Treat Your Own Spinal Stenosis

by
Jim Johnson, PT

This book was designed to provide accurate information in regard to the subject matter covered. It is sold with the understanding that the author is not engaged in rendering medical, psychological, or other professional services. If expert assistance is required, the services of a professional should be sought.

Anatomical Drawings by Eunice Johnson
Exercise Drawings by Amberly Powell

This edition published by
Dog Ear Publishing
4010 W. 86th Street, Ste H
Indianapolis, IN 46268

www.dogearpublishing.net

dog ear PUBLISHING

ISBN: 978-1-4575-4018-9
Library of Congress Control Number: Applied For
This book is printed on acid-free paper.

Printed in the United States of America

How This Book Is Set Up

- ✓ Find out exactly what the problem is and where it's at in *Chapter 1*.
- ✓ Be aware of the typical course that spinal stenosis takes in *Chapter 2*.
- ✓ Learn how you can treat spinal stenosis yourself in *Chapters 3 through 6*.
- ✓ Monitor your progress with the tools in *Chapter 7*.

Why Is The Print In This Book So Big?

People who read my books sometimes wonder why the print is so big in many of them. Some tend to think it's because I'm trying to make a little book bigger or a short book longer.

Actually, the main reason I use bigger print is for the same reason I intentionally write short books, usually under 100 pages–it's just plain easier to read and get the information quicker!

You see, the books I write address common, everyday problems that people of *all* ages have. In other words, the "typical" reader of my books could be a teenager, a busy housewife, a CEO, a construction worker, or a retired senior citizen with poor eyesight. Therefore, by writing books with larger print that are short and to the point, *everyone* can get the information quickly and with ease. After all, what good is a book full of useful information if nobody ever finishes it?

Table of Contents

1 Here's What's Going On In Your Back

After treating spinal stenosis patients for over nineteen years, I'm convinced that the first step in getting a patient better is to make sure that they have a *very* clear understanding of what it is. While some readers will no doubt open up this book *already* knowing a lot of facts about spinal stenosis, I'm betting that the majority of back and leg pain sufferers simply don't know the whole story. So without wasting any time...

The Parts of Your Spine You *Need* To Know About

I could cut to the chase and tell you that people with spinal stenosis commonly have things such as a thickened ligamentum flavum and hypertrophied facet joints, but since it's hard to even pronounce these words, much less know what they mean, it's probably best to make sure that every reader gets a little familiar with the basic structures of their back first. After that, we can then quickly move on to the *specific* changes that take place in spinal stenosis. Let's start out with the bones.

the spinal column

Most people know that their backs are made up of many small bones called *vertebrae.* Your average person has seven of them in their neck, twelve in their mid-back, and five in the lower back. I say your *average* person, because every once in awhile, I have a patient with an extra vertebra. For instance, some people might have a sixth vertebra in their lower back, instead of the usual five. On the next page, we have a picture showing each one of the vertebrae, as well as the names of the different areas of the spine that they belong to.

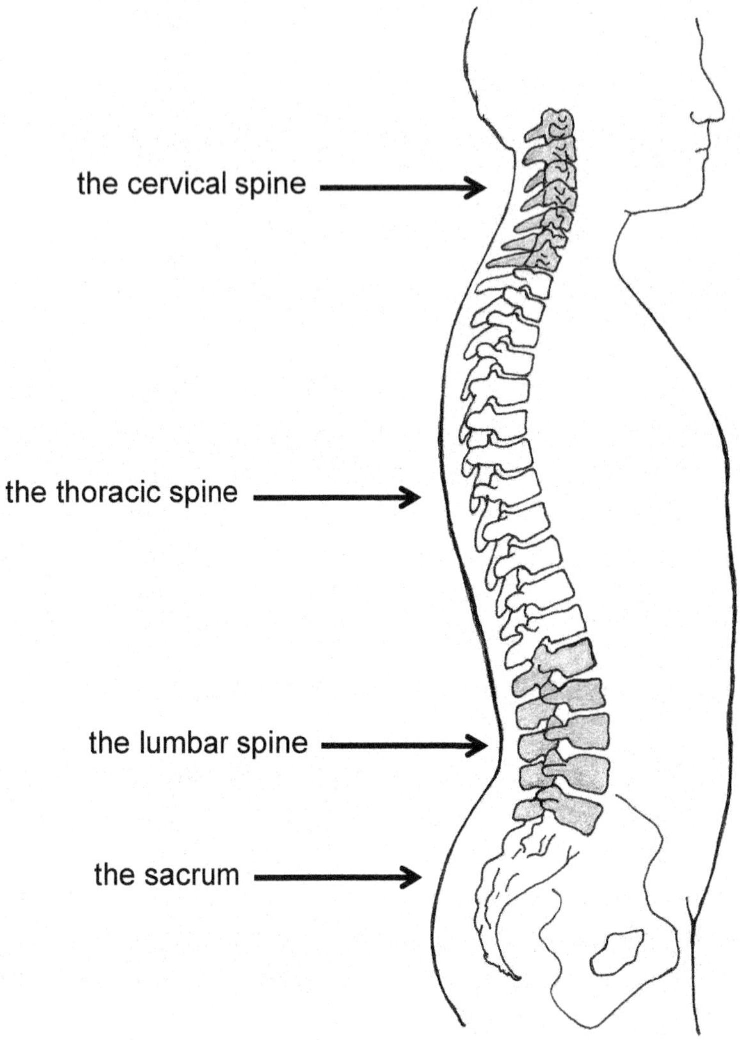

Figure 1. The bones or *vertebrae* that make up your spine.

As you can see, the vertebrae are stacked upon one another, which is what gives the spine its basic shape. Note that all twenty-four of the freely moving vertebrae are grouped into one of three main areas: the *cervical spine* (your neck), the *thoracic spine* (your mid-back), and the *lumbar spine* (your lower back). Also be aware that all the stacked vertebrae sit upon a triangular mass of fused vertebrae, known as the *sacrum*.

Okay, now that you have a general idea of how all the vertebrae bones come together to make up your spinal column, let's focus in on the one area of the spine that this book is about–spinal stenosis of the *lumbar* spine.

Now don't let "lumbar spine" confuse you–it's just some medical words that mean "lower back". The following is a close-up picture:

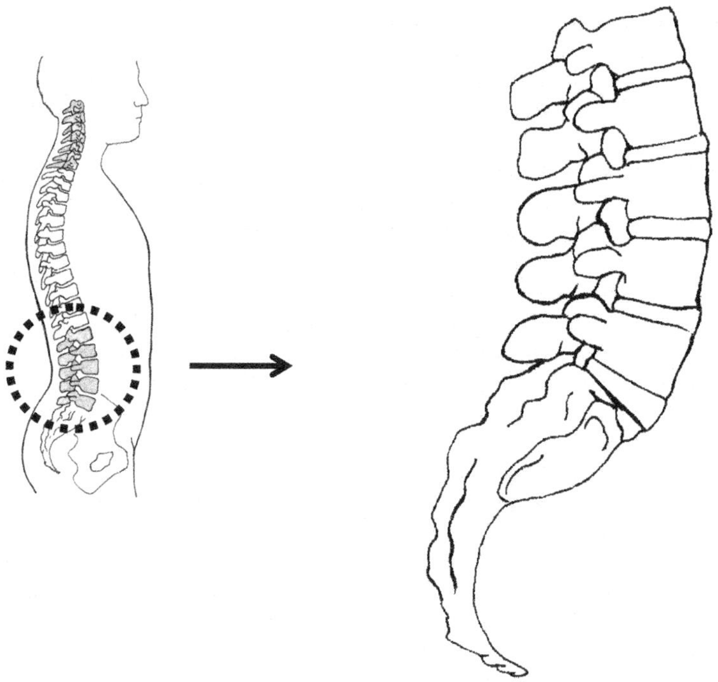

Figure 2. A sideview of the lumbar spine.

So if there's a problem with a particular vertebra in your lumbar spine, just how do doctors specify which one is which? Well, medical folks have a system. For instance, a doctor might call up another doctor and say, "I have a patient that fractured their L-2."

Talking about the vertebrae this way means that each one gets a letter (from the first letter of the area of the spine that it's from) and a number (which tells us its position starting from the top down). The following is a picture showing how each vertebrae is identified in the lumbar spine:

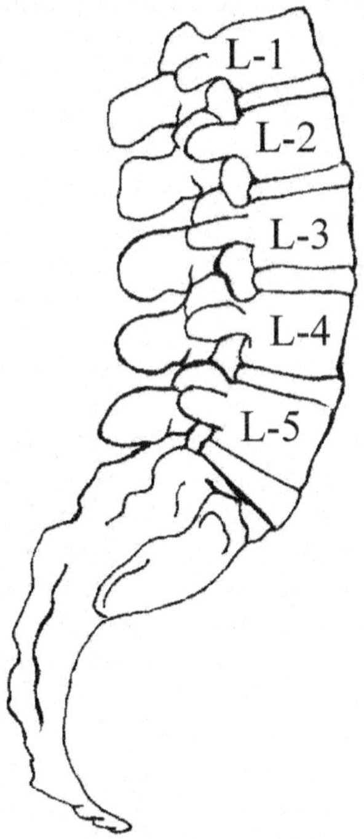

Figure 3. How the lumbar vertebrae are identified. The "L" stands for lumbar, because these vertebrae are located in the lumbar area of the spine. The number shows what position they are in, starting from the top down.

Returning to our previous example, when the doctor got a call about a patient with a fractured L-2, he knew right away that it was exactly the *second* vertebrae in the *lumbar* spine.

It's important for you too to know this information, because virtually all medical professionals use these letters and numbers when they talk about the individual vertebrae in the spine and describe what's going on. And now *you* know what they mean!

the lumbar vertebrae

As we now know, your lower back, or lumbar spine, is made up of five vertebrae. Let's pull one of them out of the stack and have a closer look at it…

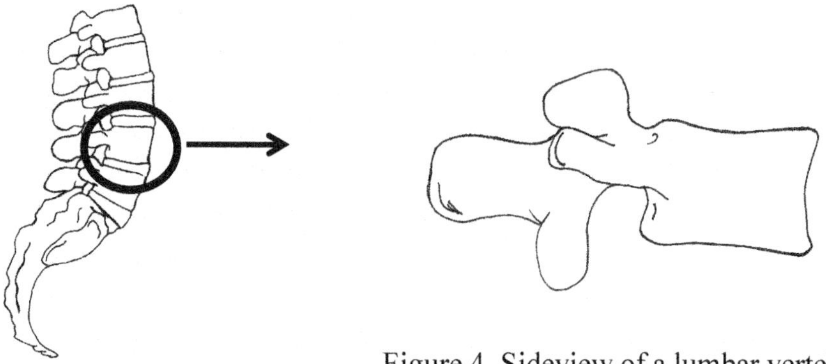

Figure 4. Sideview of a lumbar vertebrae.

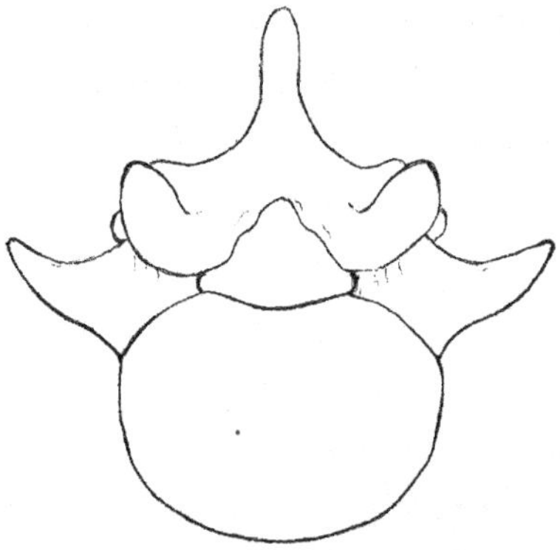

Figure 5. Overhead view of a lumbar vertebrae.

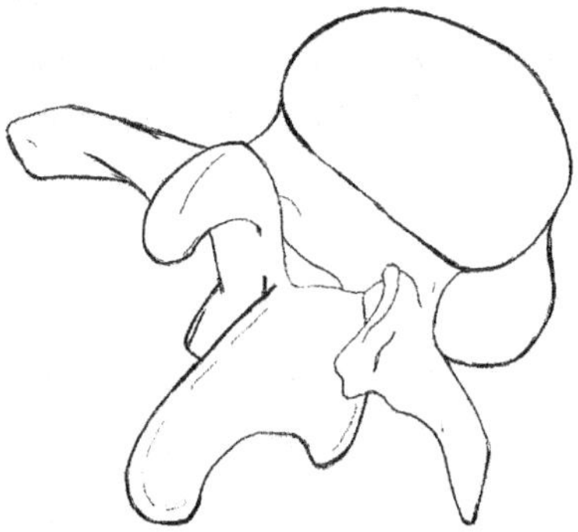

Figure 6. Angled view of a lumbar vertebrae.

Pretty odd shaped aren't they? Without going into a lot of detail, let me just say that every part you see that sticks out has *something* important that attaches to it. While they look funny by themselves, how they work becomes much clearer when you put *two* of them together…

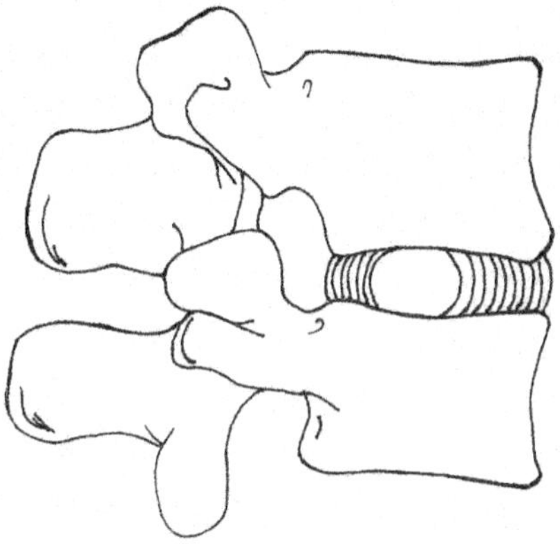

Figure 7. A close-up view of how two lumbar vertebrae fit together.

Hey, what's that thing in the middle of the two vertebrae? Well, when two vertebrae come together, the two bones aren't just shoved right up against each other, there's what's known as an *intervertebral disc* that fits in between them. Since intervertebral disc is kind of a long word, let's just call it "the disc" from here on out. Now if we take a disc out and look at it, this is what we'd see:

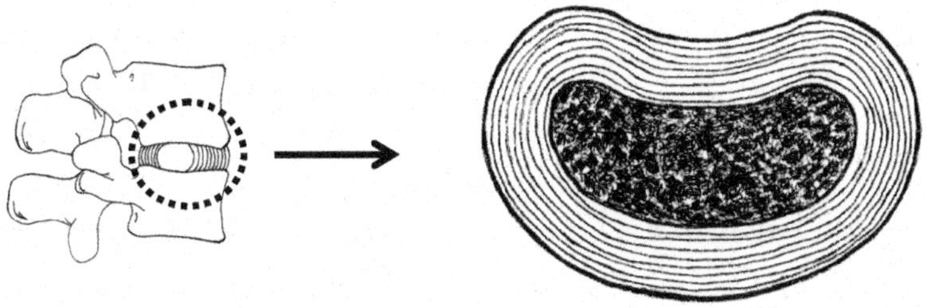

Figure 8. Looking at the disc from the top down.

You can easily tell that the middle of the disc looks a lot different than the outer layer. This is because each disc has two basic parts, the outer rings, known as the *annulus fibrosus*, and a gel-like center, called the *nucleus pulposus*.

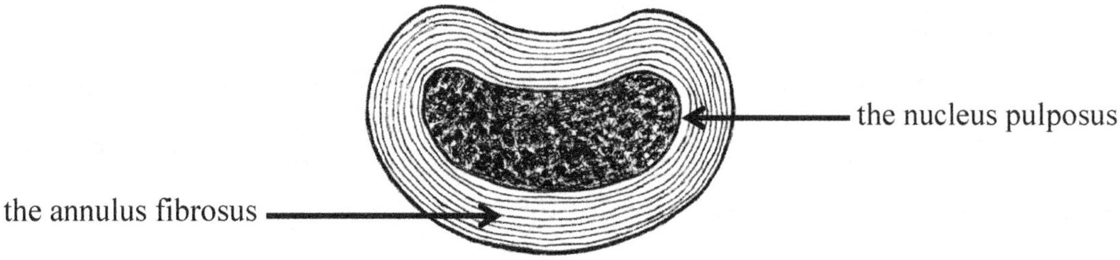

Figure 9. The two basic parts of the disc.

Have you ever heard of a "herniated disc" or a "bulging disc" or a "slipped disc"? Well, that's when the jelly-like center, the *nucleus pulposus,* has pushed into or through the rings of the annulus fibrosus. And just in case you're wondering, no, discs don't slip around!

But what do they do? Well, they don't just sit there all day doing nothing. Discs are actually *changing* their shape a bit as you bend around during the day and use your back. Here's a simple example of how the disc responds to movement and pressure:

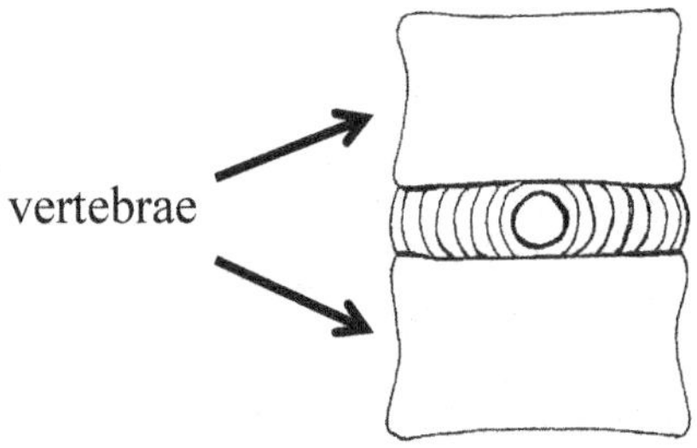

Figure 10. How the disc looks when it's not stressed.

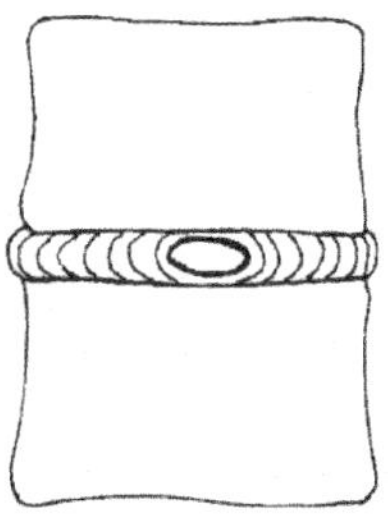

Figure 11. How the disc changes its shape when you move around and the spine is under pressure.

If any of this about the disc seems confusing to you, just think of it like a big jelly doughnut that is sitting between two bones. And if you "squish" the doughnut between the two bones, the jelly will move around. Squish it too hard too often, and it can squirt out!

the spinal joints

Now that you know that there's a disc in between your vertebrae that gives the spine a little more flexibility, another way that your vertebrae connect to each other is at the *facet joints*. Here again, don't let the medical name throw you. The facet joint is nothing more than a fancy name for the little joints in your spine.

Facet joints, like the other joints in your body, are made when two bones come together. In this case, it's the two parts of each vertebrae, known as the *articular processes,* that come together to form your spinal joints. Let's have a look at where these articular processes are located...

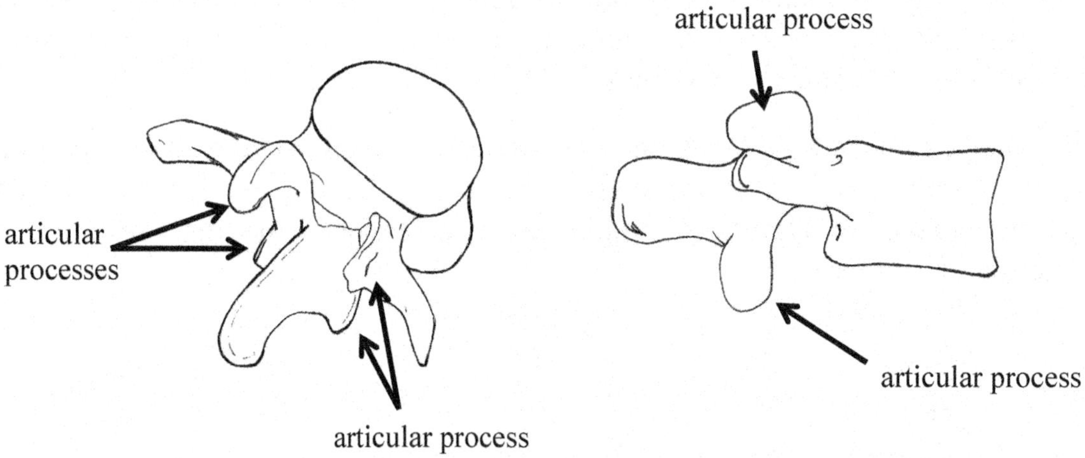

Figure 12. The articular processes of the lumbar vertebrae.

From the above pictures, you can see that each vertebrae has four articular processes, two on the upper part, and two on the bottom part.

Now that you know *where* the articular processes are, let's put together a stack of vertebrae, and see what the whole kit-and-caboodle looks like…

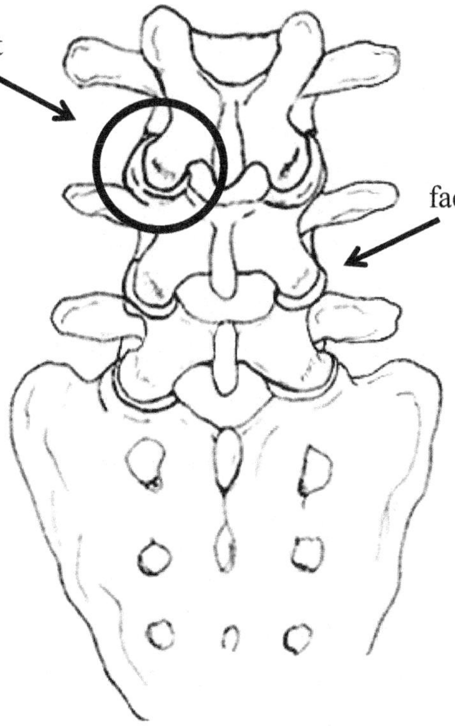

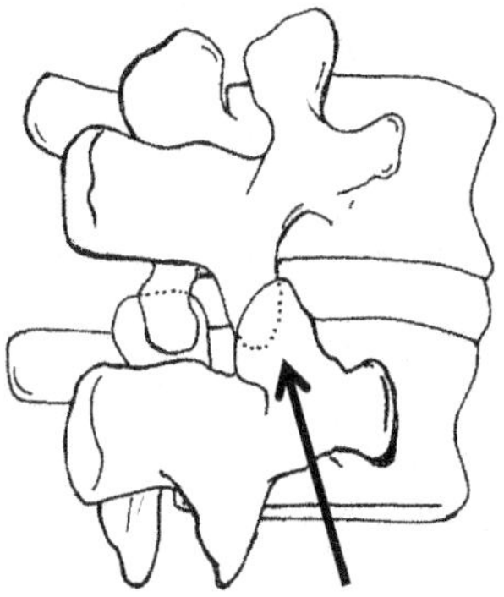

Figure 13. Looking at the lumbar spine from behind–the many pairs of tiny facet joints.

As you can see, the articular processes of each vertebrae basically "overlap" with each other when coming together to form a facet joint. *Here again, just remember that it takes two articular processes to make up one facet joint.*

Have you ever heard your back "pop" when you twisted it or had someone manipulate it? That noise occurred because the two articular processes of the facet joint were being pulled on and separated a bit. Wow!

Now a big job of the facet joints is to allow motion to occur. Here are a few pictures to give you a general idea of just how the facet joints move as you use your back:

Figure 14. How the facets joints look when you're *standing up straight*. Notice that the articular processes are in close contact with each other.

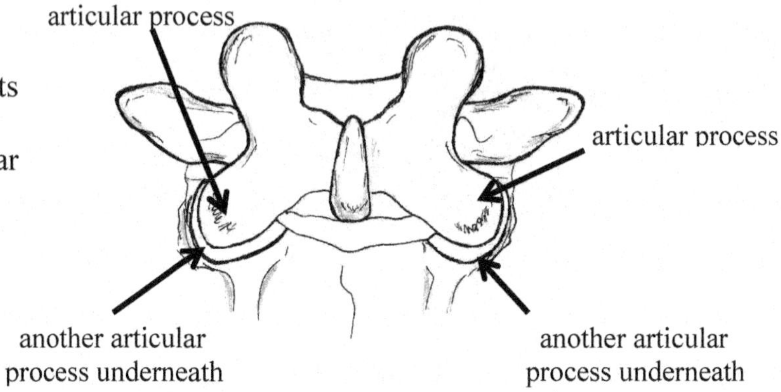

Figure 15. How the facet joints look when you're *bending forward*. Notice that the articular processes slide up.

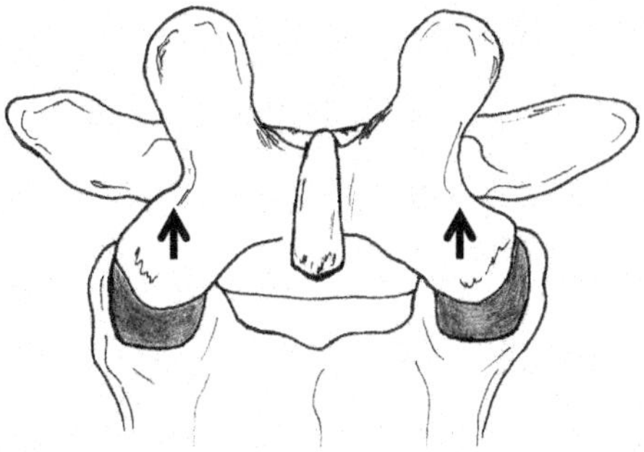

Figure 16. How the facet joints look when you *lean to the left*. Notice how much the articular process on the *right* has slid up.

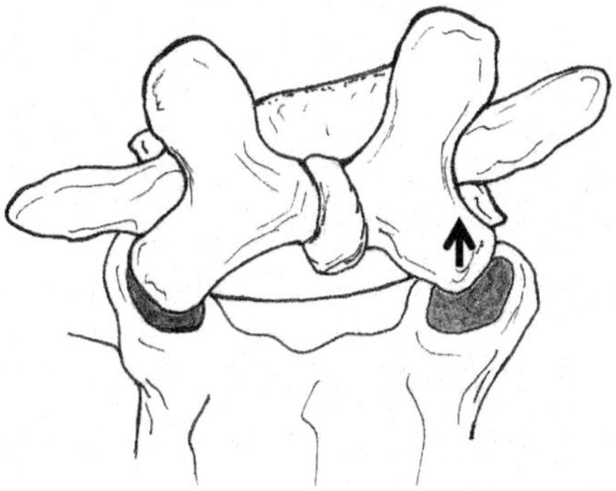

Pretty neat the way that all works, huh? Well, that about covers the major parts of your spine you need to be familiar with. Now that you have a general idea of what's what, I can finally tell you about the specific changes that are going on in a back with spinal stenosis…

Where The Problems Are in Your Back

Spinal stenosis. You can pretty much figure out what the "spinal" part means, but what's this "stenosis" word mean? Well, simply put, stenosis is when something is narrowed or becomes smaller. So if you put it all together, one gets the idea that *something* in the spine is narrowed. But what? Why is that a problem? And what causes it? This section will answer these three questions.

the two holes…and what's in 'em

While I could get all technical, by far the easiest way to tell you what is narrowed in spinal stenosis, is just to say that you have two "holes" in and around your bony spinal column–and that's where the problems are. Now the first "hole" that can become smaller, is known as your *central canal*, and it contains your spinal cord. Since there's nothing like a good picture to explain things…

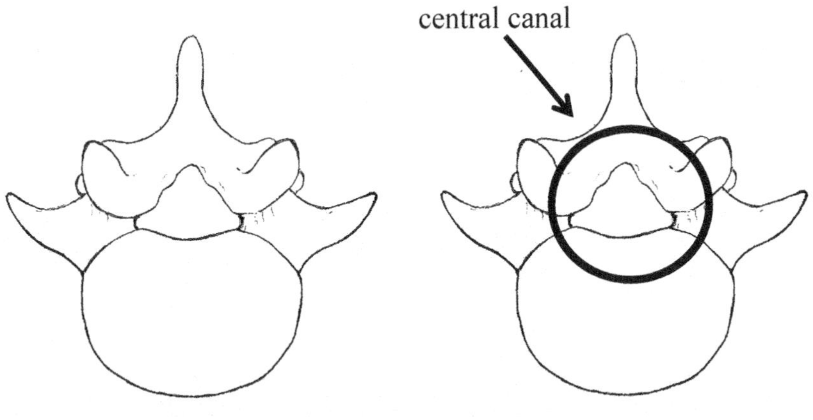

Figure 17. Looking from the top down at a lumbar vertebrae–the *central canal* which contains the spinal cord.

And the second hole? It's more on the side. This time I'll need *two* vertebrae to show you…

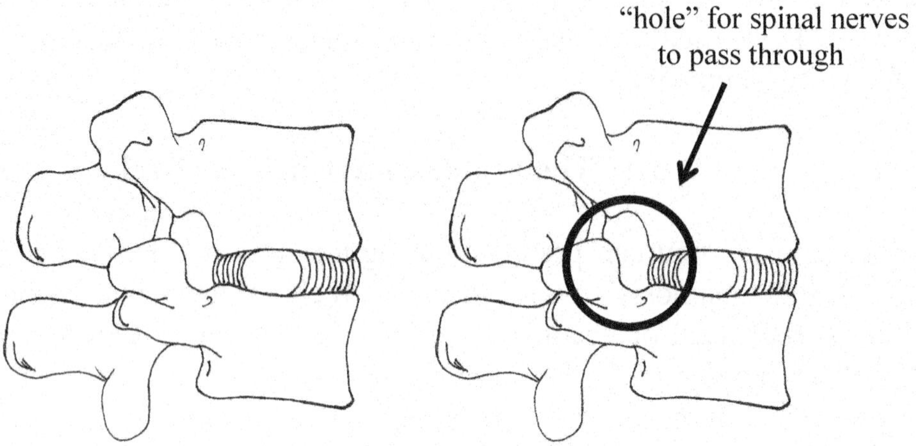

Figure 18. Looking at two lumbar vertebrae from the side. Together they form a "hole" where the spinal nerves travel through.

So now you know the answer to the first question this section set out to answer, "What in the spine is narrowed?" Spinal stenosis is when there is a narrowing of the "holes" where your spinal cord and spinal nerves pass through. As for the second question, "Why is that a problem?" this narrowing can become a problem when *too much* narrowing puts pressure on the nerves and interfere with their functioning. On to the final question, "What causes it?"

what makes the holes smaller

By far, most cases of spinal stenosis are caused by *wear and tear* of the spine over time. While there are many changes that can take place in a back, there are a few parts of it that commonly become a problem. The first change I'd like to talk about is that which occurs with the disc.

Recall that your discs are built kind of like a jelly doughnut and that they change shape as you move around and use your back. The main problem that occurs with the discs is that they tend to lose their "plumpness" over time and thin out. This would be all good and fine, except that when the discs become less plump, the two vertebrae they sit in between *come closer together*–which causes the hole on the side to become smaller! Take a look at these pictures and you'll see what I mean...

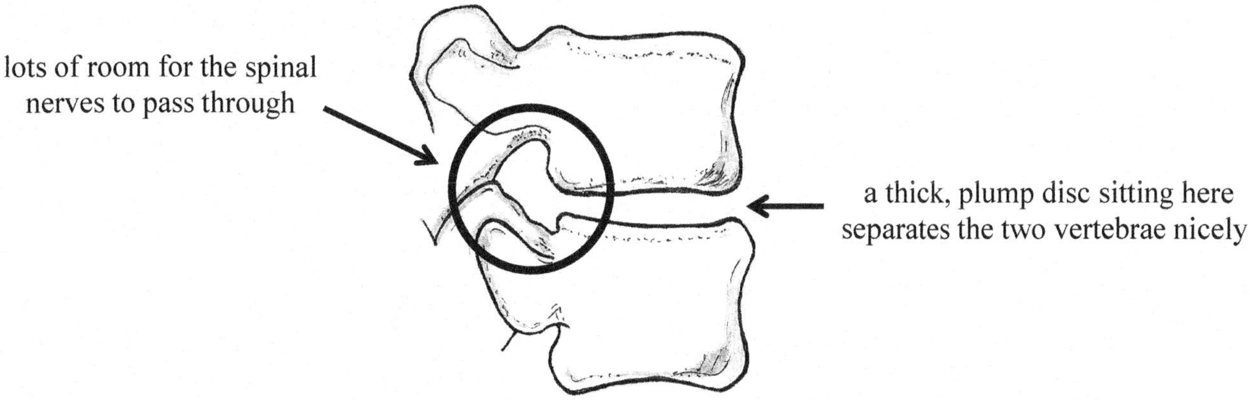
lots of room for the spinal nerves to pass through
a thick, plump disc sitting here separates the two vertebrae nicely

Figure 19. Looking at two lumbar vertebrae from the side. Look how big the "hole" is when there is a lot of space between the two vertebrae.

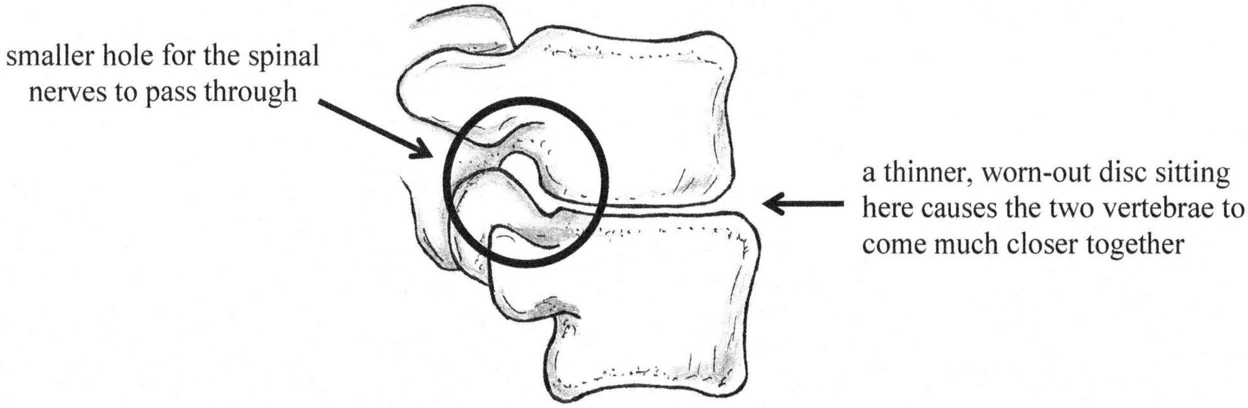
smaller hole for the spinal nerves to pass through
a thinner, worn-out disc sitting here causes the two vertebrae to come much closer together

Figure 20. As the disc becomes thinner and less plump, this causes the two vertebrae to come closer together–which makes the hole smaller! And a smaller hole could irritate the spinal nerves.

Unfortunately, the story doesn't end there. When the two vertebrae start getting closer to each other as a result of disc thinning, not only does this make the hole on the side smaller, *but it also puts extra stress on the facet joints.* And when there's too much stress on the facets, well, they react by getting *bigger* over time!

Now sometimes the facets can enlarge even before there are disc problems, but either way, the point here is that bigger facets take up more space and cause more narrowing as these pictures reveal…

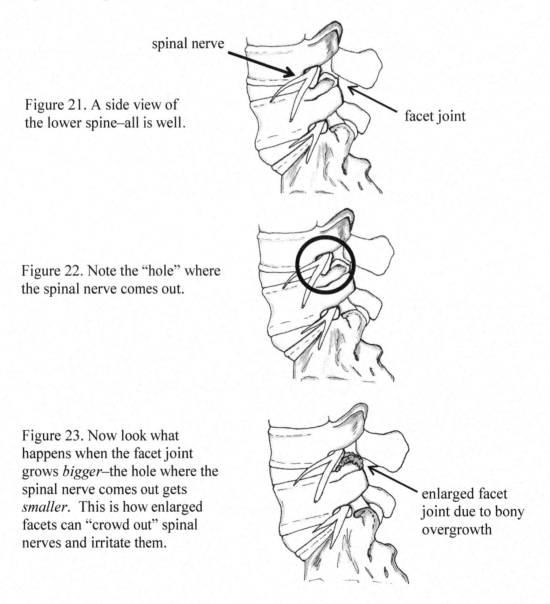

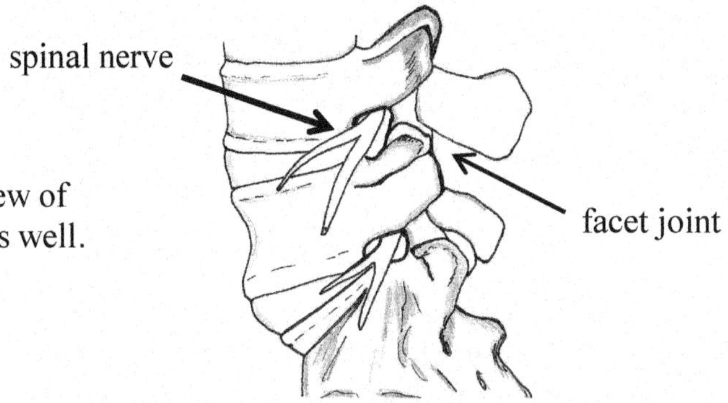

Figure 21. A side view of the lower spine–all is well.

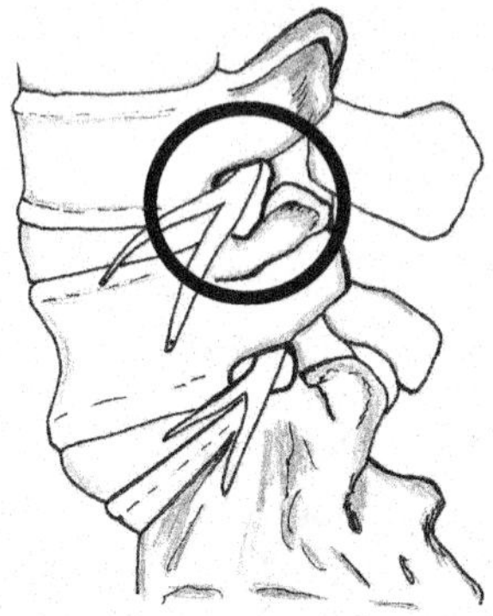

Figure 22. Note the "hole" where the spinal nerve comes out.

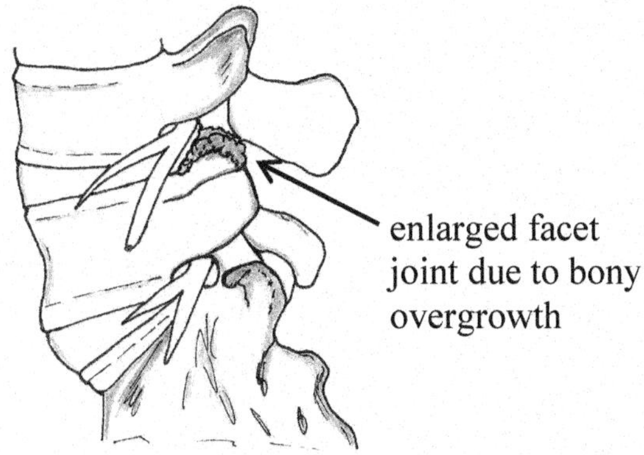

Figure 23. Now look what happens when the facet joint grows *bigger*–the hole where the spinal nerve comes out gets *smaller*. This is how enlarged facets can "crowd out" spinal nerves and irritate them.

The last common structural change we'll talk about that takes place in the back with spinal stenosis has to do with one of its ligaments. Not to be confused with tendons, ligaments are made up of a tough tissue and have the job of holding the bones together.

While there are many different ligaments in your back, the one called the *ligamentum flavum* is the most notable when it comes to spinal stenosis. Running up and down the *inside* of your central canal, here's a basic picture of where it is located:

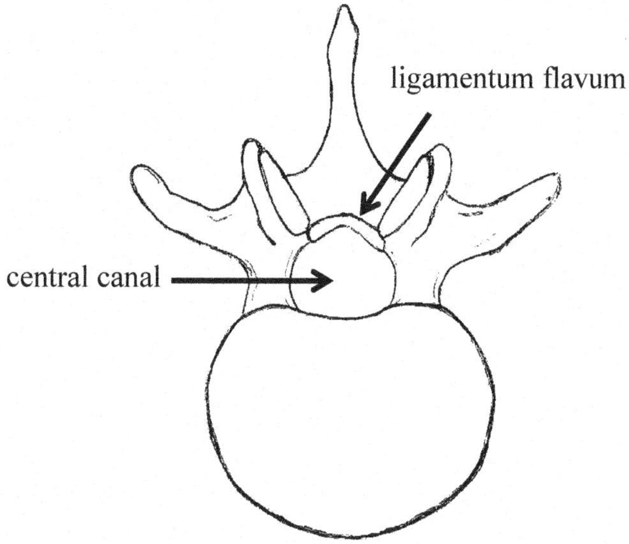

Figure 24. Looking at a lumbar vertebrae from the top down. Notice that the ligamentum flavum is located in the hole where the spinal cord sits.

The main problem that happens with this ligament, is that it becomes thicker. And this of course means that it now takes up *more* space in the central canal where your spinal cord sits–which could put pressure on it. On the next page is a series of pictures showing how a thickened ligamentum flavum can crowd out the spinal cord.

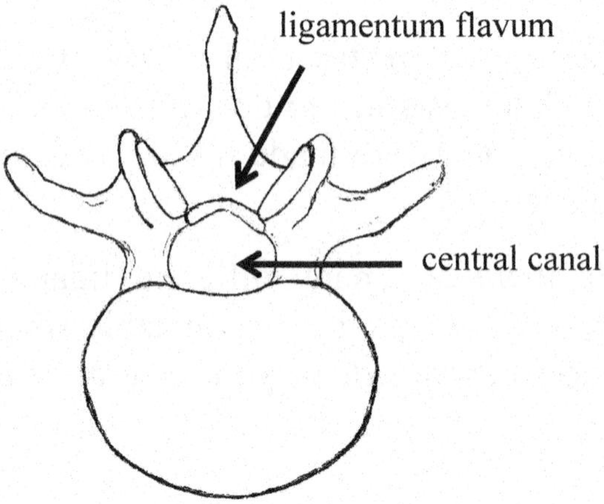

Figure 25. A normal ligamentum flavum and central canal.

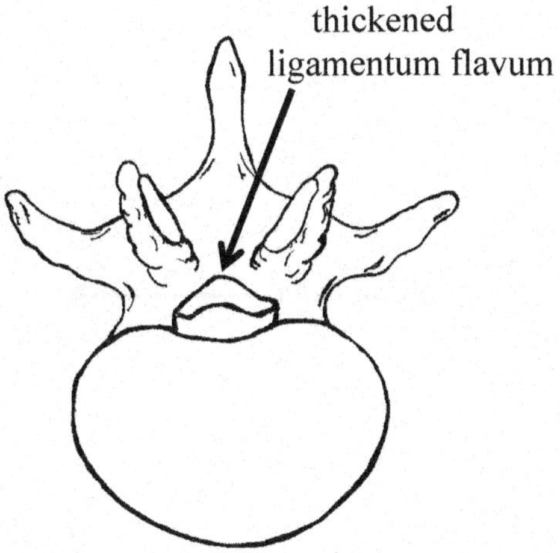

Figure 26. A thickened ligamentum flavum.

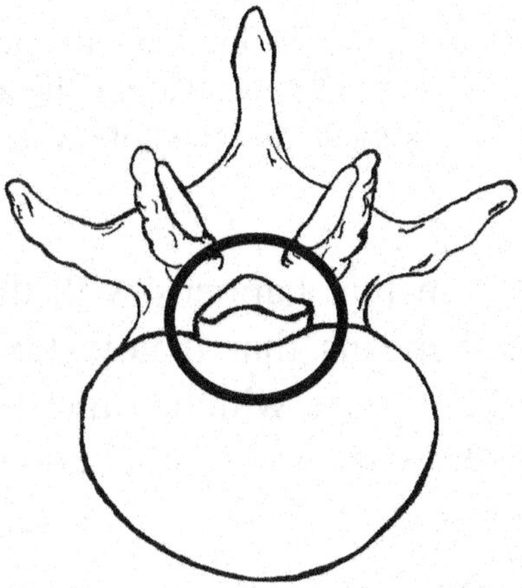

Figure 27. Notice how much smaller the central canal is with a thickened ligamentum flavum–compared to figure 25.

The Sequence of Events That Lead to Spinal Stenosis

Now that you're familiar with *what* has changed in your spine, it's time to talk about *how* these changes happen. But how can one figure this out?

Well, it's kind of like if you wanted to learn how houses are built. A good start would be to go to a new housing development and take a look around. Walking around, you would no doubt be able to see many houses in their various stages of completion–and thus get a good idea of how the finished ones got to be that way.

It's in a similar fashion that back researchers have been able to get a good idea of the changes that lead to spinal stenosis. Just like observing a new housing development, scientists have closely examined large numbers of autopsy specimens of the lumbar spine of all different ages (Kirkaldy-Willis 1978). And based upon such observations, scientists have then been able to piece together the sequence of events that lead to spinal stenosis.

Now there are a couple of different ways you can look at the whole process. The first one looks at the development of spinal stenosis from an anatomical or "nuts and bolts" point of view. It goes something like this:

- the changes that lead to spinal stenosis typically begin with the disc (Butler 1990). Discs have a tendency to get less plump as we age, and injuries can also make the disc break down to varying degrees over time.

- as the disc starts to get less plump, the vertebrae get closer to each other (see Figures 19 and 20). This throws more stress than normal on the facet joints, which in turn causes them to get bigger over time (see Figure 23). The ligamentum flavum also gets thicker as a result of the abnormal stresses in the area (see Figure 26).

- all these changes, the disc getting thinner, the facet joints getting larger, and the ligaments getting thicker, all narrow the holes where the spinal cord and spinal nerves pass through–and thus create spinal stenosis.

The other way of describing the sequence of events that lead to spinal stenosis, is to think about it in terms of how much *motion* there is in the spine at the various points of the process. Looking at spinal stenosis this way, scientists have found three distinct stages that go something like this...

- problems for the spine begin in the **dysfunction stage**, as the disc begins to lose its plumpness due to aging and injury. Researchers looking at spine specimens that are in this stage, usually see tears in the disc and irritation of the facet joints.

- this leads to the **instability stage**. Now that the disc has lost some of its plumpness and is starting to get thinner, the vertebrae begin to move closer to each other. This in turn throws abnormal stresses on the facet joints, *causing the vertebrae to start moving around excessively and become unstable to varying degrees.* Researchers looking at spine specimens in this stage, typically see facet joints that move too much (increased laxity) and find discs that are becoming pretty disrupted on the inside.

- last comes the **stabilization stage**. As a result of enlarged facet joints, and bony overgrowths called *osteophytes,* the vertebrae actually *lose* motion and start to become stable once again.

- now once the vertebrae at a particular level of the spine stiffen up and lose motion, this throws *more* stress on the vertebrae directly *above* it. This increased stress eventually wears down the above vertebrae and disc, and the whole process tends to repeats itself. This is how spinal stenosis can spread from one level of the spine to the next one above it–eventually affecting many different levels of your back.

When I explain spinal stenosis this way to patients, most are interested in the fact that the spine can actually stabilize itself over time. And how exactly does that happen? Well, basically through the extra growth that takes place in various areas. For instance, I've shown you pictures of enlarged facet joints, so you can probably can get a good idea of how a bigger, irregularly shaped joint with worn down surfaces would tend to stiffen up. Remember those pictures on page 10 which shows how the facet joint moves by sliding up and down? Just imagine how hard it would be for the bones to slide up and down properly if the joint surfaces became rough!

Yet another major reason things stiffen up over time, are due to these things I mentioned earlier called *osteophytes*. Osteophytes are little overgrowths of bone that many people know as bone spurs. They form in response to increased stress and excessive motion in an area–especially at the edges of the discs in your spine.

So what do they look like, and how do they limit motion? The following series of pictures tells the tale...

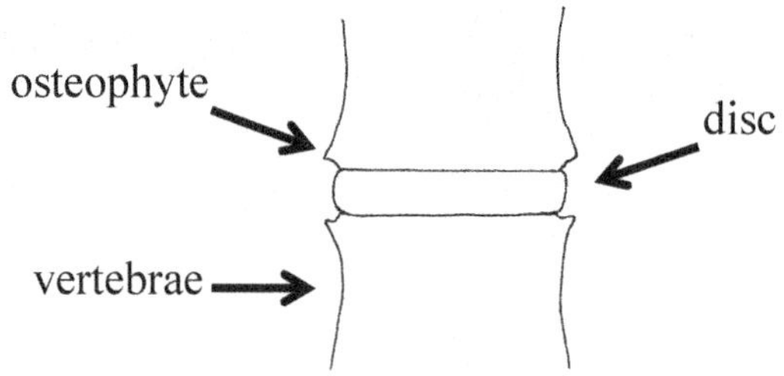

Figure 28. Side view of a disc in between two lumbar vertebrae. Osteophytes are just starting to form.

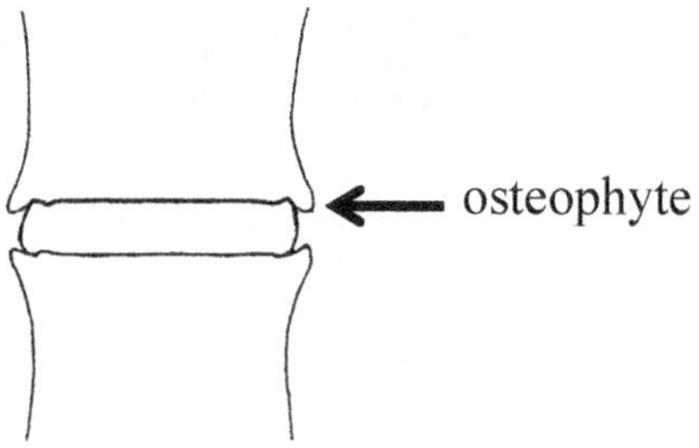

Figure 29. The osteophytes continue to grow in response to excessive tension on the disc and extra motion in the vertebrae.

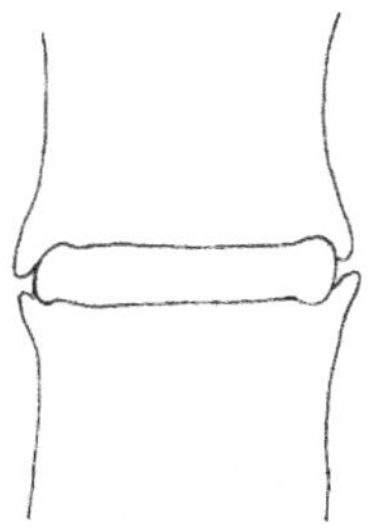

Figure 30. As the extra stress and tension continues, the osteophytes grow even more.

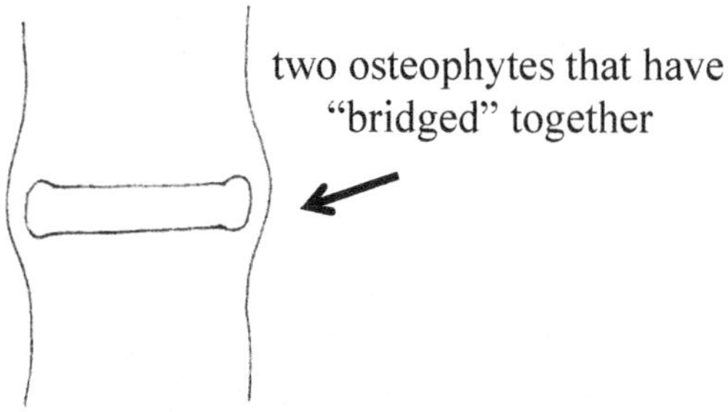

Figure 31. Over time, osteophytes can actually "bridge" together–which stabilizes the vertebrae and greatly limits spinal motion.

So any way you look at spinal stenosis and describe the whole process, the main thing to keep in mind is that the narrowing that occurs is caused by a *series* of specific changes in your spine. And these changes all occur in response to certain stresses that your back is subjected to over time.

Why You Are *Not* Doomed

While this chapter has been informative, I'm sure there are many readers that are getting pretty discouraged at this point. I mean after all, I've shown you picture after picture of enlarged joints, sharp bony spurs, and narrowed holes in your vertebrae just waiting to crowd out your spinal nerves. Some might even be thinking, "My back is a mess, there's no way I can *ever* get better!"

Well, I'm here to tell you that you are *not* doomed. The reason I can say this is simply because there are many people walking around with the very changes I've been describing in this chapter, *and have no pain.* Put another way, it's quite possible to have spinal stenosis in your back and feel just fine.

How can I say such a thing with any kind of confidence? By looking at the research that has been done on people with *no* back pain. Let's have a quick look at a few studies and you'll see what I mean…

- one study took 67 people with *no* back pain or sciatica and scanned their low backs with an MRI (magnetic resonance imaging). In the group that was 60 to 80 years old, 21% had spinal stenosis (Boden 1990).
- yet another study used MRI and looked at 33 people over fifty-five years of age. All had *no* symptoms. What did they find? 69% had at least *mild* central canal stenosis, 29% had at least *moderate* central canal stenosis, and 6% had *severe* central canal stenosis (Tong 2006).
- in this study, MRI scans were done on 31 people with *no* back pain between the ages of fifty-five and eighty years old. 23% had spinal stenosis (Haig 2007).

At this point, some readers may be skeptical and find this hard to believe. After all, spinal stenosis puts pressure on the nerves so you'd *have* to have some pain, right? Yet another popular misconception. Check out these studies…

- this one looked at 300 *asymptomatic* individuals who had myelograms. A myelogram is an x-ray study where dye is injected into the spine which outlines the spinal cord and nerve roots. This in turn enables doctors to see if there's any pressure on things. The researchers found that 24% of subjects showed some type of nerve compression in their low back (Hitselberger 1968).
- another study took 46 volunteers with *no* back pain and examined them with an MRI. 21% of them had something either touching or pressing on a nerve in their back (Boos 1995).
- researchers in this study did MRI scans on 60 people *without* back pain. Interestingly, 22% of subjects had something touching a spinal nerve, 7% had something pressing on a nerve enough to displace it, and 2% showed actual compression of a nerve. (Weishaupt 1998).

The moral of the story is this. Of course spinal stenosis can be painful and cause many nasty symptoms–on this you'll get no argument from me. *But,* it's also possible to have spinal stenosis, even *severe* spinal stenosis, and have no pain at all–many studies published in peer-reviewed journals like the ones above have clearly shown this. Furthermore, you can also have pressure or compression on spinal nerves *without* having any pain.

So the question now is, why do some people with spinal stenosis have symptoms and others don't? What makes the difference?

Well, we don't have *all* the answers yet, but new research is giving us clues. For instance:

- researchers compared a group of 28 people who had spinal stenosis and pain, to a group of 16 people who had spinal stenosis and *no* pain (Yagci 2009). A test which can check the electrical activity of the back muscles, called an electromyogram (or EMG), was done on both groups, as well as MRI scans of their low back. It was found that 93% of the subjects with spinal stenosis and pain showed abnormalities in their back muscles with EMG testing. On the other hand, 94% of the patients with spinal stenosis and *no* pain had *normal* back muscles with EMG testing.

Apparently there are *other* problems going on in spinal stenosis than just the structural abnormalities we see pictured all so clearly on X-rays and MRI scans. In the above study, you wouldn't have been able to tell which group had pain based on their MRI's because both group's pictures showed all the changes that go along with spinal stenosis. *However you would be able to tell which group had pain if you looked at whose back muscles were working the best!*

And where does *that* leave us? Well, for one, in a lot more optimistic position. In this book, we're not going to be concerned with trying to change things such as enlarged facet joints, narrowed holes or thickened ligaments. We know from many studies that it's *quite* possible for people to live just fine with these kinds of changes–so we're going to let them be.

So what are we going to focus on? *Improving the function of your back.* Why? Because functional problems, like improperly working back muscles, seem much more related to one having pain, than how bad pictures of your spine look on an MRI. Therefore, this book is going to lead you step-by-step through a series of "tune-ups" that are specifically designed to get your spine in good working order. If you've got weak back muscles, we're going to get them stronger. If your back is stiff, well, we're going to loosen it up–and so on.

The game plan is sound. Pain is the result of something not functioning properly–so if we improve the functioning of your back, your symptoms will also improve. I've been using this principle with patients for over nineteen years now, and as you'll soon see, we have some pretty good studies that show it *really* works!

Quick Review

- ✓ **your low back, or *lumbar spine*, is made up of five vertebrae**
- ✓ **a disc, which is put together like a jelly doughnut, sits between the vertebrae**
- ✓ **tiny joints, called the facet joints, help connect the vertebrae together and allow the spine to move**
- ✓ **there are two main "holes" in and around your spine where the spinal cord and nerves pass through**
- ✓ **spinal stenosis is when these "holes" start to narrow and become smaller–which can put pressure on your spinal cord and nerves**
- ✓ **the process of spinal stenosis usually starts when the disc becomes less plump as a result of injury and aging–which brings the vertebrae closer together**
- ✓ **when the vertebrae get closer together, this throws abnormal stresses on the facet joints, and causes them to break down and become unstable. An important ligament, known as the ligamentum flavum, also thickens as a result of increased stress in the area.**
- ✓ **the whole process of spinal stenosis typically goes through three stages: a dysfunction stage, an instability stage, and a stabilization stage**
- ✓ **studies show that people can have spinal stenosis and nerve compression and still have *no pain***
- ✓ **it's easier to distinguish people with painful spinal stenosis from people who have non-painful spinal stenosis by looking at functional things such as how well the back muscles are working–rather than how images of the spine look on an MRI**
- ✓ **this book treats spinal stenosis symptoms by improving the functioning of your back**

2 What Will Happen to Your Back Over the Long Run?

It's the question that's on the mind of most people with spinal stenosis: "What's going to happen to my back over the long run?"

Scientifically speaking, the only way to know for sure what typically happens to people with spinal stenosis over time, is to conduct what is called a *natural history study*. Natural history studies attempt to find out exactly how long a disease (or problem) will last on its own, naturally, without interference, by following a group of patients over time that receive *no medical treatment.*

Problem is, it's tough to get together a group of people with spinal stenosis, give them no treatment, and then just sit back and watch them for a few years! About the closest study you'll find like this in the medical literature on spinal stenosis went something like this:

Study #1

- 32 people with spinal stenosis were just observed for an average of 49 months, or about 4 years (Johnsson 1992)
- lumbar myelogram showed a complete block in 13% of subjects
- nobody had surgery, and the study didn't specify that the patients got any treatment in particular
- four year follow-up showed that symptoms in 70% of the patients were unchanged, improved in 15%, and got worse in 15%
- no proof of severe deterioration was found after four years

What I didn't like about this study was the fact that we don't really know for sure what kind of treatment the patients got, if any. However that aside, this study does bring spinal stenosis sufferers some good news. It shows us that it isn't the case at all that everybody with spinal stenosis is doomed to get worse over time. In fact, 70% remained stable over the four year observation period *and 15% even improved.* Apparently it's far from being a given that all the changes in your spine that cause narrowing continue in a downhill spiral.

Other studies have also shown optimistic results. For instance, one decided to tackle things another way. Instead of just looking at one group of people with spinal stenosis, and follow them for awhile, these researchers decided to observe *two* groups of patients…

Study #2

- researchers got together a group of 54 people with spinal stenosis (Herno 1996). They had surgery.
- researchers then got together another group of 54 people with spinal stenosis *that were matched to the first group* by their age, sex, major symptoms, myelogram findings, and duration of symptoms. This group had no systematic conservative treatment, such as physical therapy.
- notably, there were some people in each group that had either a total or subtotal block on their lumbar myelogram
- both groups were followed for an average of four years
- results from the four year follow-up showed that there were no differences in the outcome between the two groups

Here again, it's nice to know that you can have spinal stenosis, and still do well *without* resorting to surgery. But what about if you try conservative therapy, such as exercise, and it doesn't work? Will you end up worse in the end because you delayed having the back surgery that you should have had awhile ago? Well, let's take another look at the research...

Study #3

- 100 subjects with spinal stenosis were given either surgery or conservative treatment (Amundsen 2000)
- patients were followed for 10 years
- more than half of the conservatively treated patients had a satisfactory outcome
- over the 10 year study, some patients in the conservative therapy group ended up having back surgery
- at the 10 year follow-up, researchers concluded that surgery for spinal stenosis was equally beneficial whether a person had it right away, or if they waited for several years

Seems there is no harm done in delaying spinal stenosis surgery–because those who chose to wait awhile to have it ended up doing just as well as those who went under the knife right off away.

I think this is a really good study to know about, because some readers might be sitting here wondering if they should really be having back surgery instead of reading a book about treating spinal stenosis on their own. Now you know.

Okay. We've answered some important questions so far, but we still haven't tackled the big one, namely, "Does spinal stenosis *ever* go away?"

A crucial question, and since the title of this chapter is "What Will Happen to Your Back Over the Long Run", let's answer it here and now. I know of only one study that has done a technically good enough job to provide us with some meaningful information. Here's how it went...

Study #4

- researchers in this study observed 32 subjects with spinal stenosis who were between the ages of 55 and 80 years old (Haig 2006)
- all subjects underwent MRI's of the lumbar spine
- none chose surgery, and conservative treatments were not described in the study
- researchers followed patients for an average of 20 months, or just over a year and a half
- long-term follow-up showed improvements in spinal anatomy, with 6 subjects showing an *increase* in spinal canal diameter

This is a very notable observational study. It's my favorite kind, a prospective study, meaning that researchers followed the patients *forward* over time, as opposed to retrospective, where they simply look *back* in time, at say, some medical records. While I wish the follow-up period would have been for more years, it still makes a extremely promising point: it's not a given at all that spinal stenosis patients get worse over time, and in fact, some actually end up with less stenosis!

Now after reading all these study results, I don't want you to get the wrong impression. I am *not* saying that *all* spinal stenosis patients get better over time and that it goes away. Obviously there are some people with spinal stenosis that need surgery because they are losing muscle strength quickly, or have a decline in their bowel and bladder function.

Instead, what I'm saying, is that the literature clearly shows us that a rapid or catastrophic neurologic decline is actually *rare* in spinal stenosis patients. And in reality, there are many scientific studies published in peer reviewed journals that have shown the tendency for many patients with spinal stenosis to actually *improve* over time–*with conservative treatment.*

Hmmm. So the million dollar question is, if it's been shown that many spinal stenosis sufferers can actually get *better* and improve their symptoms with conservative treatment, which treatments work the best?

Well, the studies we've just gone over don't really give us many specific answers in that department–however there are other studies that do. And that's exactly what the remainder of this book is all about: the best treatments to improve spinal stenosis symptoms in the shortest amount of time–*that you can do all on your own.*

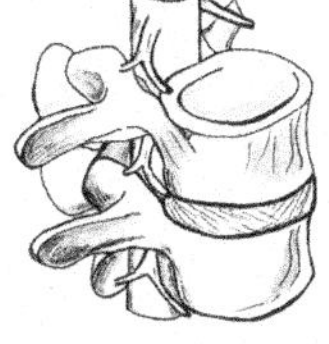

Quick Review

- ✓ **there are no true natural history studies to tell us what will happen to spinal stenosis patients over the long run when it goes untreated**
- ✓ **there are, however, some observational studies that can give us some clues**
- ✓ **a good number of scientific studies have shown us that when spinal stenosis patients are followed for years and treated conservatively (without surgery), many actually improve**
- ✓ **it has also been shown that a rapid or catastrophic neurologic decline is rare in patients with spinal stenosis**
- ✓ **according to long-term studies, delaying surgery and trying conservative therapy does *not* give you a poorer prognosis over the long run**

3 Tune-Up #1: How to Make Your Back *Much* Stronger

The first thing we're going to tune-up is your back muscles. But why? How do we even know there's anything wrong with the back muscles of people who have spinal stenosis?

Well, for one, there's that study we talked about at the end of Chapter 1. If you recall, it went like this:

- researchers compared a group of 28 people who had spinal stenosis and pain , to a group of 16 people who had spinal stenosis and *no* pain (Yagci 2009). A test which can check the electrical activity of the back muscles, called an electromyogram (or EMG), was done on both groups, as well as MRI scans of their low back. It was found that 93% of the subjects with spinal stenosis and pain showed abnormalities in their back muscles with EMG testing. On the other hand, 94% of the patients with spinal stenosis and *no* pain had *normal* back muscles with EMG testing.

So from that study, we know that abnormalities in the back muscles do indeed exist in people with spinal stenosis. And it's also a good way of telling apart who with spinal stenosis as seen on MRI has pain–and who doesn't. Which is all a clear indication that we need to get those back muscles working better! Other studies poking around the back muscles of people with spinal stenosis have found similar things:

- researchers performed EMG's on the back muscles of 22 patients who had spinal stenosis (Leinonen 2003)
- 18 of the 22 patients had abnormalities in their back muscles

As these last two studies point out, not everyone with spinal stenosis has a problem with their back muscles, but the majority do–and it's definitely something we need to address.

Make Sure You Strengthen *This* Back Muscle

If you notice in these studies, I've been saying that researchers have found abnormalities in "the back muscles". What I've left out, is that they've really found most of the problems with *one* muscle in particular. Which one? It's called the *multifidus*.

If you've never heard of the multifidus (pronounced "mull-TIFF-i-dus"), you're not alone. A lot of medical professionals, including many doctors I have treated, also look at me funny when I talk about the multifidus. And to be completely honest, the multifidus wasn't significant to me either until I graduated from physical therapy school and started having a special interest in low-back problems. Since the multifidus is probably a mystery muscle to most people, let's start out by looking at a picture of it...

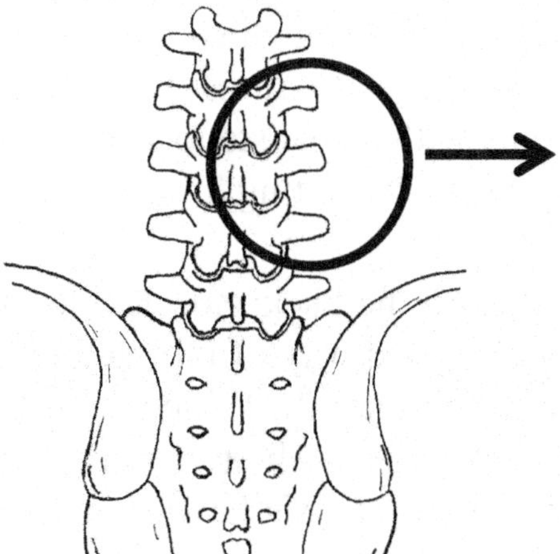

Figure 32. Looking at the lumbar spine from the back.

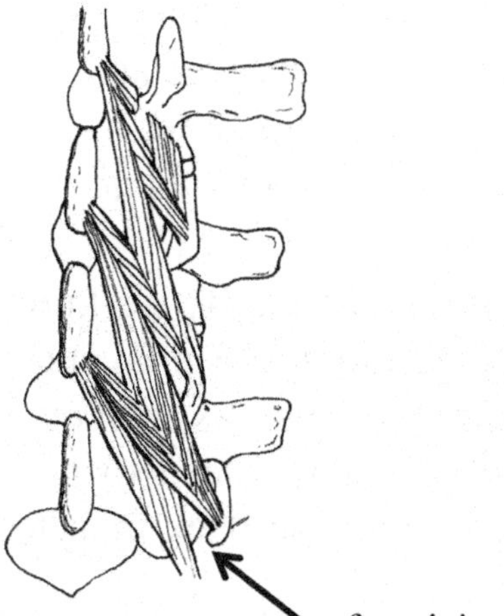

Figure 33. The multifidus muscle.

As you can see, the multifidus is really kind of a group of muscles, but since it's referred to in the back literature in the singular, I'll be calling it "the multifidus" as well.

Now the multifidus is just one of your many back muscles. The name comes from the Latin words *multus*, meaning many, and *findo*, to cleave. Looking back at Figure 33, you can see how early anatomists might have come up with such a name.

Back muscles are arranged on the spine in several layers, with the multifidus being on of the more deeply situated ones. The multifidus muscle group starts out in the lower back and runs the entire length of the spine, all the way up to your neck. However it's not just one big muscle that runs all the way from the top to the bottom. Instead, it takes many individual multifidus muscles combined, each crossing *two to five* levels of vertebrae, to cover the entire spinal column. In this way, the multifidus is capable of gaining fine control over just a single segment of the spine. This anatomic detail is important to know, because researchers are now finding out that in some people with back pain, it's not always the whole multifidus muscle group that's the problem–sometimes it's just a *single* multifidus at only *one* level of the spine that's not working properly.

Now muscles need nerves to carry a signal to them in order to make them contract and relax. Think of a nerve like an electrical cord that carries power to a lamp to make it light up. The multifidus is no different in that it also needs nerves to function. However what makes it different from the other back muscles, is that each multifidus muscle gets its nerve messages from only *one* level of the spinal cord. Anatomists call this being *segmentally innervated.* What this means to the multifidus muscle is that it can be more prone to having problems. Other back muscles have their nerves or "electrical cords" coming from several different levels of the spine to power them, so that if one nerve doesn't work well, it still has others to help it out. The multifidus, however, doesn't have it so easy, as its nerve supply comes from just a single level of the spine. Therefore, if something does go wrong at a certain level in the spine, such as when something presses on a nerve, a single multifidus muscle could be in big trouble without a backup!

Another interesting anatomic fact about the multifidus is that it's connected to each of the facet joints in your spine by way of its attachment to the joint capsule (the tissue that surrounds the joint). This is significant for the spine's function, because it's part of the job of the multifidus to contract with certain back movements and help pull the capsule away from the joint so it won't be nipped. A multifidus that isn't working properly has the potential to allow this capsule to be pinched by the joint. Since it's an anatomical fact that the capsule has nerve endings, any pinching of it can result in an attack of back pain. This might help explain some of the strange cases of back pain attacks people complain of after doing seemingly simple motions they do every day, such as sweeping a floor. If the joint is caught off guard, and the multifidus muscle is unable to control things–ouch!

One can already begin to see, just by this short discussion of anatomy alone, how an abnormal multifidus not doing its job properly has great potential to create a lot of back problems. Also makes you wonder what gives you the most trouble–an abnormal multifidus found in many people with painful spinal stenosis, or the abnormal structural changes found in many people with pain*less* spinal stenosis…

How to Find The Multifidus Muscle on Yourself

Want to find this problem muscle on yourself? Well, the last picture showed us that the multifidus runs up and down the spine, but it's really much thicker in the low back region at your waist level. It is here you will be able to feel it directly through the overlying skin the best.

To do this, first locate the bones that stick up in the center of your back. These are called *spinous processes*, and are easily felt because they are the only ones that stick out in the middle and run up and down your back. Once you have felt these bones, feel directly off to the side of one of them in your low back (either side will do), and you should feel a soft mass of tissue….which are some of your multifidus muscles! It is here that they sit nicely in a groove on each side of the spinous process bones that stick up.

Know that as you move farther *up* the spine, it will become much harder to feel just the multifidus by itself. This is because the muscles of the back are arranged in layers, and as you feel your way up towards the head from waist level, other back muscles will soon begin to overlap and cover up the multifidus muscle. This in effect "buries" the multifidus at higher levels of the back, which makes it less accessible and impossible to feel by itself. You can, however, be confident that you are feeling *just* the multifidus muscle under the skin at the beltline level in your lower back area.

So how do *your* multifidus muscles feel? Normal muscles feel soft, and almost spongy-like. And usually your fingers will be able to go quite easily through the overlying skin and superficial fat, sinking down into the muscle tissue without feeling much resistance. *On the other hand*, muscles that are overworked or irritated for one reason or another can sometimes go into spasm, feeling firm or even very hard. When patients come to see me, they will often times describe their back muscles by saying that they feel "knots" in their back. These kinds of things will limit the overall function of a muscle, making its job harder or even impossible to do.

Now keep in mind that a little tenderness here and there is okay, depending on how hard you're pressing, but no muscle should really be that painful in its normal state.

What the Multifidus Does

So what exactly does a funny looking muscle like the multifidus do anyway? Well, to answer this question, we have to look at two rather specific areas to get a complete picture of its job in the back. The first is the study of kinesiology, where one looks at things such as the angle that a muscle can pull on a bone. The other area? EMG studies, which can tell us how active a muscle is during certain movements of the spine. Let's take a brief look at each…

the kinesiology of the multifidus muscle

Don't let the word "kinesiology" fool you. It's just a big word that means the study of how things move. You can see from this definition that we need to know a little bit about kinesiology in order to fully understand what the multifidus does.

Basically, just think of muscles like rubber bands that are stretched from one bone to another. When muscles receive a signal by the nerves to contract, they then pull on the bones they're attached to. And, like a stretched rubber band, they become shorter in length. This then causes the bone that the muscle is pulling on to move. It's in this manner that we are able to move our bones, and in turn, our arms and legs. Now that we have this knowledge, we can use it to figure out what the job of the multifidus is.

Looking back at the picture of the multifidus on page 32, you can see that it attaches to the backside of your vertebrae. This clue tells us that the muscle pulls the vertebrae or spine backwards, since a rubber band stretched this way over the back of two bones could only pull them in this direction. Therefore, just looking at where the muscle is placed in the back, and the direction it pulls in, one can see that *the multifidus is responsible for a backward tilting effect on each of the individual vertebrae in the spine.*

EMG of the multifidus muscle

So now we know what the multifidus can do as it pulls on two vertebrae bones in your back–however this doesn't really tell us the *whole* tale. Sure we know that it pulls the vertebrae backwards, but when does it do this, and with what motions? Well, this is where the study of electromyography, or EMG comes in pretty handy.

An EMG study starts when a muscle is hooked up to a machine that can tell us when the muscle is active and working. The machine can do this by recording the electrical activity of the muscles a person uses them.

When I first started studying the multifidus in the early 90's, I went straight to the medical library to find all the research articles I could get my hands on that studied the multifidus muscle with an EMG machine. I was glad to find that there was indeed much literature published in medical journals through the years that had studied the back muscles with an EMG machine as people performed certain movements or exercises. According to these studies, your multifidus *is* active and working when you are…

- standing still
- bending forward
- twisting to either side
- picking or lifting things up
- walking

On the other hand, I also found out that your multifidus is *not* active or working when you are…

- sidebending the back directly to the left or right
- bending backwards when there is no resistance
- laying down

You can see from these lists that your multifidus is a *very* busy back muscle. In fact, the available research shows us that this muscle is involved in the vast majority of movements and activities that we do with our spines every day. But wait a minute–didn't we just look at the kinesiology of the multifidus and find out that all it does is pull the vertebrae backwards in a rocking type of motion? Indeed it does, but obviously this motion is a very important while the spine is moving in various ways. Otherwise, it wouldn't be as highly active as it is with so many back motions!

a proven stabilizer of the back

Having good stability in your back means that the back is able to keep itself in positions that are safe. When the back loses this control, even momentarily, motion can take place in positions that could potentially cause damage to its structures. For example, say you're putting away a heavy bowl on a high shelf, a little to the right, which causes you to stretch and slightly twist your low back. The back that has good stability will be able to keep its vertebrae, joints, and discs within a safe zone and be able to control its motion well. Additionally, it has the ability to hold odd positions better for a longer period of time. On the other hand, a back that has poor stability is unable to control motion well and could let the spine exceed its zone of safety–thereby risking injury. Interestingly, your spine has several ways of keeping itself safe and stable…

- with *passive* structures, such as ligaments, joints, bones, etc.
- with *active* structures, which are the muscles which actively contract

While both the active and passive elements contribute to the stability of the back, some things have been shown to provide more support than others. Research on back stabilization has demonstrated that the human spinal column without muscles is unable to support normal loads that we place on it during everyday activities. This tells us that the passive structures, like ligaments, bones and discs are, in and of themselves, quite incapable of supporting the spine. And so, the muscles stand out as a major source of stability for our backs. But which one have scientists found to be the most important? I'll give you three guesses– although I'm sure all you need is one.

Yes, it's true. While all the muscles in the back have the ability to support and stabilize the spine, the multifidus has emerged from the research as being able to contribute more stability than the rest. Here are several facts from what the back research has uncovered about the multifidus that pinpoints it as being a *key* stabilizer of the spine…

- the multifidus is capable of providing control over *individual* segments of the spine
- when it contracts, the multifidus can stiffen the vertebrae, and in turn, the individual levels of the spine, thereby providing support and stability
- about 2/3 of the total stiffness that all the back muscles can provide for support through muscle contraction comes from the multifidus!

A properly functioning back is one that has good support *and* can keep itself from being injured. As you can see, the spine relies quite heavily on its muscles for this job. And of all the muscles in the back, the research identifies *the multifidus* as having the biggest role of all in providing this necessary stability and control.

The *Correct* Way to Get Your Multifidus in Shape

Okay. Now that you know all about a small muscle that's a big problem in spinal stenosis, it's time to learn how to make it *stronger*.

But before jumping right in and going over all the exercises you'll ever need to beef up your multifidus, I think it's best to begin with a few strength training basics. Because I wrote this book with *everyone* in mind–from the bodybuilder who lifts hundreds of pounds, to the retired person who just wants to be able to pick up their grandkids–it's only wise to make sure that we're all on the same page before going any further. Then, when we do get down to describing each of the strengthening exercises, *every* reader will know exactly what I mean when I say, "Do 1 set of 20 reps." So, using the handy question and answer format, let's start at the beginning...

How do we make a muscle stronger?

Muscles get stronger only when we constantly challenge them to do more than they're used to doing. Do the same amount and type of activity over and over again, and your muscles will *never* increase in strength. For example, if Karen goes to the gym and lifts a ten-pound dumbbell up and down, ten times, workout after workout, week after week, her arms will *not* get any stronger by doing this exercise. Why? Because the human body is very efficient.

You see, right now, Karen's arm muscles can already do the job she is asking them to do (lift a ten-pound dumbbell ten times). Therefore, why should they bother growing any stronger? I mean after all, stronger, bigger muscles *do* require more calories, nutrition and maintenance from the body. And since they can *already* do everything they're asked to do, increasing in size and demanding more from the rest of the body would only be a waste of resources for no good reason.

It makes perfect sense if you stop and think about it, but we can also use this same line of thinking when it comes to making our muscles bigger and stronger–we simply *give* them a reason to get into better shape. And how do we do that? By simply asking them to do *more* than they're used to doing. Going back to the above example, if Karen wants make her arm muscles stronger, then she could maybe switch from a ten-pound dumbbell to a *twelve*-pound dumbbell the next time she goes to work out. Whoa! Her arm muscles won't be ready for that at all–they were always used to working with that ten-pound dumbbell. And so, they will have no choice but to get stronger now in order to meet the new demand Karen has placed on them.

For the more scientific minded readers, the physiology textbooks call this *progressive resistance exercise.* You can use this very same strategy to get *any* muscle in your body stronger, and we're certainly going to be using it to get your multifidus as strong as we can.

What's the difference between a repetition and a set?

As we've said, we need to constantly challenge our muscles in order to force them to get stronger and one good way to do this is to lift a heavier weight than we're used to using. Of course you won't always be able to lift a heavier and heavier weight *every* time you do an exercise, and so another option you have is to try to lift the same weight *more* times than you did before. As you can see, it's a good idea to keep track of things, just so you know for sure that you're actually making progress–which is where the terms "set" and "repetition" come into play.

If you take a weight and lift it up and down over your head once, you could say that you have just done one repetition or "rep" of that exercise. Likewise, if you take the same weight and lift it up and down a total of ten times over your head, then you could say that you did ten repetitions of that exercise.

A set, on the other hand, is simply a bunch of repetitions done one after the other. Using our above example once again, if you lifted a weight ten times over your head, and then rested, you would have just done one set of ten repetitions. Pretty straightforward isn't it?

Now the last thing you need to know about reps and sets is how we go about writing them down. The most common method used, is to first write the number of sets you did of an exercise, followed by an "x", and then the number of repetitions you did. For example, if you were able to lift a weight over your head ten times and then rested, you would write down 1x10. This means that you did 1 set of 10 repetitions of that particular exercise. Likewise, if the next workout you did 12 repetitions, you would write 1x12.

What's the best number of sets and repetitions to do in order to make a muscle stronger?

There was a time when I asked myself that same question. So, in order to find out, I completely searched the published strength training literature starting from the year 1960. I then sorted out just the randomized controlled trials, since these provide the highest form of proof in medicine that something is really effective, and laid them all out on my kitchen table. While getting to that point took me literally months and months of daily reading and hunting down articles, it was really the only way I could come up with an accurate, evidence-based answer.

Now the first conclusion I came to was that it is quite possible for a person to get significantly stronger by doing any one of a *wide* variety of set and repetition combinations. For instance, one study might show that one set of eight to twelve repetitions could make a person stronger compared to a non-exercising control group, but then again so could four sets of thirteen to fifteen reps in another study.

Realizing this, I decided to change my strategy a bit and set my sights on finding the most *efficient* number of sets and repetitions. In other words, how many sets and repetitions could produce the best strength gains with the least amount of effort? And so, I had two issues to resolve. The first one was, "Are multiple sets of an exercise better than doing just one set?" and the second, "Exactly how many repetitions will produce the best strength gains?

Anxious to get to the bottom of things, I returned once again to my pile of randomized controlled trials, this time searching for more specific answers. Here's what I found as far as sets are concerned:

- there are *many* randomized controlled trials showing that *one* set of an exercise is just as good as doing *three* sets of an exercise (Esquivel 2007, Starkey 1996, Reid 1987, Stowers 1983, Silvester 1982). This has been shown to be true in people who have just started weight training, as well in individuals who have been training for some time (Hass 2000).

Wow. With a lot of my patients either having limited time to exercise or just hating it altogether, that was really good news. I could now tell them that based on strong evidence from many randomized controlled trials, all they needed to do was just *one set* of an exercise to get stronger–which would get them every bit as strong as doing three!

And the best number of repetitions to do? Well, that wasn't quite as cut and dried. The first thing I noted from the literature was that different numbers of repetitions have totally different training effects on the muscles. You see, it seems that the lower numbers of repetitions, say three or seven for example, train the muscles more for *strength.* On the other hand, the higher repetition numbers, such as twenty or twenty-five, tend to increase a muscle's *endurance* more than strength (endurance is where a muscle must repeatedly contract over and over for a long period of time such as when a person continuously moves their arms back and forth while vacuuming a rug for several minutes).

Another way to think about this is to simply imagine the repetition numbers sitting on a line. Repetitions that develop strength sit more toward the far left side of the line, and the number of repetitions that develop mainly endurance lie towards the right. Everything in the middle, therefore, would give you varying mixtures of both strength and endurance. The following is an example of this:

The Repetition Continuum

1 rep	10 reps	around 20 reps and higher
strength ———————————	———————————	endurance ——————→

Please note, however, that it's not like you won't gain *any* strength at all if you do an exercise for twenty repetitions or more. It's just that you'll gain mainly muscular endurance, and not near as much strength than if you would have done fewer repetitions (such as five or ten).

Okay, so now I knew there was a big difference between the lower repetitions and the higher repetitions. However one last question still stuck in my mind. Among the lower repetitions, are some better than others for gaining strength? For example, can I tell my patients that they will get stronger by doing a set of three or four repetitions as opposed to doing a set of nine or ten?

Well, it turns out that there really is no difference. For example, one randomized controlled trial had groups of exercisers do either three sets of 2-3 repetitions, three sets of 5-6 repetitions, or three sets of 9-10 repetitions (O'Shea, 1966). After six weeks of training, everyone improved in strength, *with no significant differences among the three groups.*

And so, with this last piece of information, my lengthy (but profitable) investigation had finally come to an end. After scrutinizing some 45-plus years of strength training research, I could now make the following evidence-based conclusions:

- doing one set of an exercise is just as good as doing three sets of an exercise
- lower repetitions are best for building muscular strength, with no particular lower number being better than the others
- higher repetitions (around 20 or more) are best for building muscular endurance

In this book, we'll be taking full advantage of the above information by doing just one set of an exercise for ten to twenty repetitions. This means that you will use a weight that you can lift *at least* ten times in a row, and when you can lift it twenty times in good form, it's time to increase the weight a little to keep the progress going.

And why did I pick those numbers? Two reasons. The first has to do with the job of the multifidus. Since its role is primarily that of a stabilizer, we want to boost its endurance and a long holding time the most. And this means we're going to lean a little more towards the *upper* repetitions in order to boost the endurance ability of the multifidus, while still staying low enough to substantially increase its strength. Remember, from around the twenty repetitions mark and up, you're going to gain mostly muscular endurance and a lot less strength.

The second reason? Well, it's a matter of safety. Using higher repetitions enables us to not only gain plenty of strength, but also use much *lighter* weights than if we'd chosen to work with the lower repetitions. This is because it takes a much heavier weight to tire a muscle out in, say, five repetitions, than it does to tire a muscle out in fifteen. And since most people would agree that you have a better chance of injuring yourself with a heavier weight as opposed to a lighter one, I recommend leaning more towards the upper repetitions.

How many times a week do I have to do the exercises?

Doing the same strengthening exercise every day, or even five days a week will usually lead to overtraining–which means *no* strength gains. This is because the muscles need time to recover, which typically means at least a day or so in between exercise bouts to rest and rebuild before you stress 'em again. And so, the question then becomes, which is better, one, two or three times a week?

Well, believe it or not, when I went through the strength training literature in search of the optimal number of times a week to do a strengthening exercise, there were a few randomized controlled trials actually showing that doing a strengthening exercise *once* a week was just as good as doing it two or three times a week. However, these studies were done on *very* specific populations (such as the elderly) or *very* specific muscle groups that were worked in a special manner. Therefore, when you take this information, and couple it with the fact that there are a few randomized controlled trials showing that two and three times a week are far better than one time a week, there really isn't much support for the average person to do a strengthening exercise once a week to get stronger. And so, we're again left with another question of which is better, two versus three times a week–which is what much of the strength training research has investigated.

However it is at this point that the waters start to get a little muddy. If you take all the randomized controlled trials comparing two times a week to three times a week and lay them out on a table, you will get mixed results. In other words, there are some studies showing you that doing an exercise two times a week will get you the *same* results as three times a week, **but** there's also good research showing you that three times a week is *better* than two times a week. So what's one to do?

Well, in a case like this, the bottom line is that you can't really draw a firm conclusion one way or the other. So, you've got to work with what you've got. In this book, I'm going to recommend that you shoot for doing the strengthening exercises *three* times a week, because there is some good evidence that three times a week is better than two times a week (Braith 1989). However, I'm also going to add that if you have an unbelievably busy week, or just plain forget to do the exercises, I'll settle for two times a week because there is also substantial evidence that working out two times a week is just as good as working out three times a week (Carroll 1998, DeMichele 1997).

So there you have it. While it may have been a whole lot easier to just answer the question by saying "do the strengthening exercise two to three times a week," I think it's good for readers to know *exactly* why they're doing the things I'm suggesting *and* that there's a good, evidence-based reason behind it.

How hard should I push it when I do a set?

How hard you push yourself while doing an exercise, also known as *exercise intensity*, is another issue that certainly deserves mention and is a question I am frequently asked by patients. The answer lies in two pieces of information:

1. Doing an exercise until no further repetitions can be done in good form is called *momentary muscular failure*. Research shows us that getting to momentary muscular failure or close to it produces the best strength gains.
2. You should not be in pain while exercising.

Taking the above information into consideration, I feel that a person should keep doing an exercise as long as it isn't painful and until no further repetitions can be done in good form within the repetition scheme.

Does it make any difference how fast you do a repetition?

Many randomized controlled trials have shown that as far as gaining strength is concerned, it does *not* matter whether you do a repetition fast or slow (Berger 1966, Palmieri 1987, Young 1993). Here's a look at one of the studies:

- subjects were randomly divided into three groups (Berger 1966)
- each group did one set of the bench press exercise, which was performed in 25 seconds
- the first group did 4 repetitions in 25 seconds, the second group did 8-10 repetitions in 25 seconds, and the third did 18-20 repetitions in 25 seconds
- at the end of eight weeks, *there were no significant differences in the amount of strength gained between any of the groups*

So that's as far as strength is concerned. As far as safety, I recommend that you lift the weight up and down *smoothly* with each repetition, carefully avoiding any jerking motions.

The Key Exercises For a Stronger Back

There are lots of exercises that involve the multifdus muscle and stimulate it to get stronger. But because not everybody has the same back, I can't give just one exercise hoping that it will work for every single reader of this book. This is where the process can get a little hairy, because if you were my patient, I would try out different exercises with you and find the one that works the best (yes, all you need is *one*).

But since that *isn't* possible, I will instead show you a variety of exercises that work the multifidus muscle, and then leave it up to you to try them and pick the one which works best for you. To that end, I've included one you can do on your stomach, one on your hands and knees, and one in standing.

This first series of exercises are my very first choice to give someone for multifidus strengthening. I always have patients try this one initially, as it is done with the low back in a "neutral" or middle position, and therefore has the least chance of aggravating anyone's symptoms. In the clinic, it has seemed to agree with about 90 percent of patient's backs.

Multifidus Strengthening Exercise #1

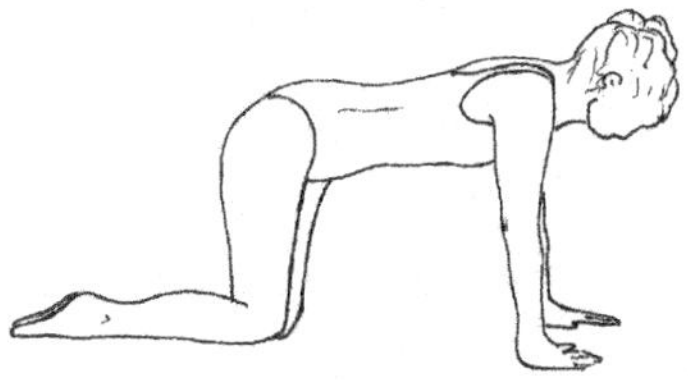

Starting Position

1. You should be on all fours.
2. Your back should be in a middle or "neutral" position (not too bent or too straight, but comfortable above all).

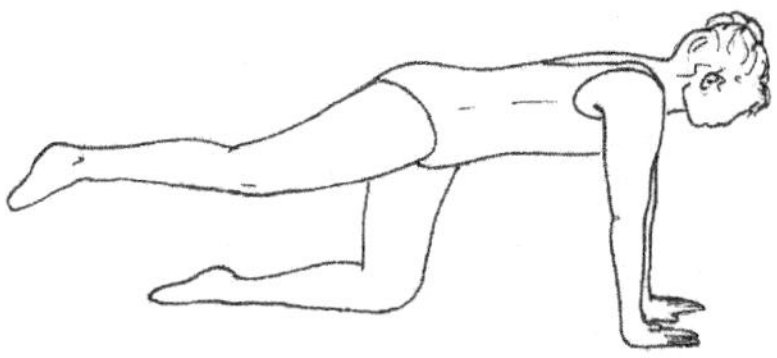

Exercise Movement

1. Raise one leg close to the horizontal, hold for a second, and lower.
2. Try not to let the lower back move while doing the exercise.
3. Repeat this sequence with the other leg.
4. Do this over and over again, *alternating* the right and left legs, eventually working up to a total of 20 repetitions *with each leg* over time.
5. Do this exercise one time a day, two to three days a week, with a day of rest in between.
6. When you can do this exercise for a total of 20 repetitions in a row *with each leg*, move on to Multifidus Strengthening Exercise #2.

The multifidus can only grow stronger if it is consistently being challenged by some sort of progressive resistance. This is what Exercise #2 does–places a bit more of a load on your multifidus by adding the weight of your arms.

Multifidus Strengthening Exercise #2

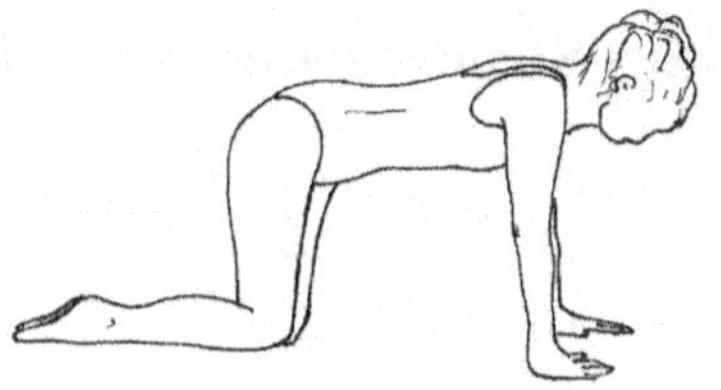

Starting Position

1. You should be on all fours.
2. Your back should be in a middle or "neutral" position (not too bent or too straight, but comfortable above all).

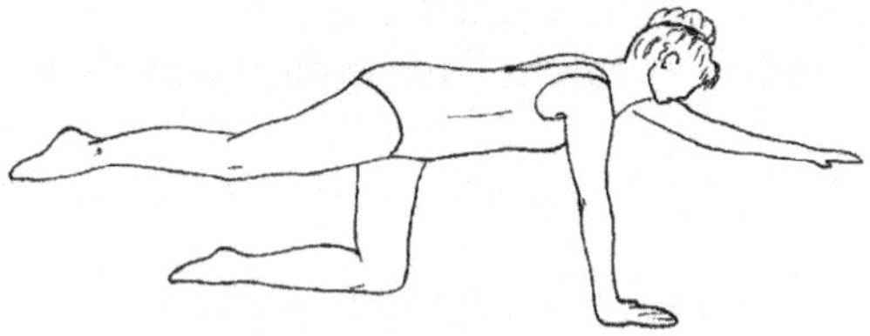

Exercise Movement

1. Raise the right leg and left arm up, close to the horizontal, *at the same time*.
2. Hold for a second, then lower them both.
3. Try not to let the lower back move while doing the exercise.
4. Repeat, except this time raise the left leg and the right arm up, close to the horizontal, at the same time.
5. Hold for a second, then lower, trying not to let the lower back move.
6. Do this over and over again, *alternating* the right leg/left arm with the left leg/right arm and eventually working up to a total of 20 repetitions over time (that would be a total of 20 with the right leg/left arm and 20 with the left leg/right arm).
7. Do this exercise one time a day, two to three days a week, with a day of rest in between.
8. When you can do this exercise for 20 repetitions in a row (a total of 20 times with the right leg/left arm and 20 times with the left leg/right arm, move on to Multifidus Strengthening Exercise #3.

This is the last exercise in this series. It's done exactly the same way as Multifidus Strengthening Exercise #2, except this time you are going to add ankle weights to further increase the load on the multifidus. How much weight should you add? Well, that depends. My guess is anywhere from a 1 to a 5 pound ankle weight on each ankle. I can't tell you exactly because I don't know how much you weigh or how strong you are. This is where you will have to be the judge. Start out with a pound or two and adjust as necessary so that you are able to do the exercise correctly *for at least 10 repetitions* or so.

Multifidus Strengthening Exercise #3

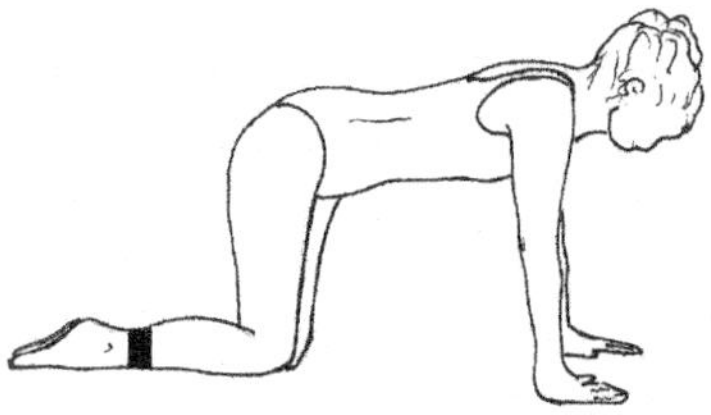

Starting Position

1. You should be on all fours.
2. Your back should be in a middle or "neutral" position (not too bent or too straight, but comfortable above all).

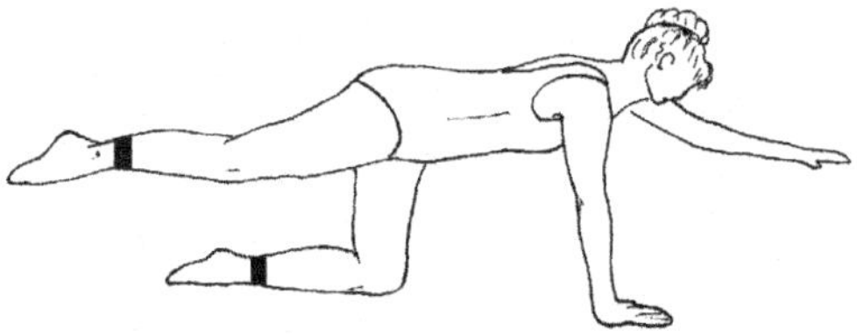

Exercise Movement

1. Raise the right leg and left arm up, close to the horizontal, *at the same time.*
2. Hold for a second, then lower them both.
3. Try not to let the lower back move while doing the exercise.
4. Repeat, except this time raise the left leg and the right arm up, close to the horizontal, at the same time.
5. Hold for a second, then lower, trying not to let the lower back move.
6. Do this over and over again, *alternating* the right leg/left arm with the left leg/right arm and eventually working up to a total of 20 repetitions over time (that would be a total of 20 with the right leg/left arm and 20 with the left leg/right arm).
7. Do this exercise one time a day, two to three days a week, with a day of rest in between.

a note on progressing and maintaining strength gains

When you have reached the point where you can do Multifidus Strengthening Exercise #3 for 20 repetitions (a total of 20 times with the right leg/left arm, and a total of 20 times with the left leg/right arm) with light ankle weights, you should have built up good strength in your multifidus muscles. Then, to maintain this strength, just do Multifidus Strengthening Exercise #3 once or twice a week using the same weight and doing the same amount of repetitions that you last did.

For example, let's say you feel your back now has good strength and you can do Multifidus Strenghtening Exercise #3 for 20 repetitions using 2-pound ankle weights on each leg. Doing Multifidus Strengthening Exercise #3 for 20 repetitions with the 2-pound ankle weights on each leg *once a week* is all that is necessary to keep your current strength levels.

On the other hand, if you feel that your back does need more strength, depending on your goals, job, activities and such, just continue to add more weight to the ankles progressively, a little at a time, until you're where you need to be.

As stated earlier, Multifidus Strengthening Exercises #1 through #3 are my number-one choice for strengthening the multifidus muscles. However, there may be a few readers who, for some reason or another, are unable to get on their hands and knees to do the exercises. That's where the next set of exercises comes in. Although they aren't my absolute first choice, they will give the multifidus a workout and succeed in strengthening it nonetheless.

Multifidus Strengthening Exercise #4

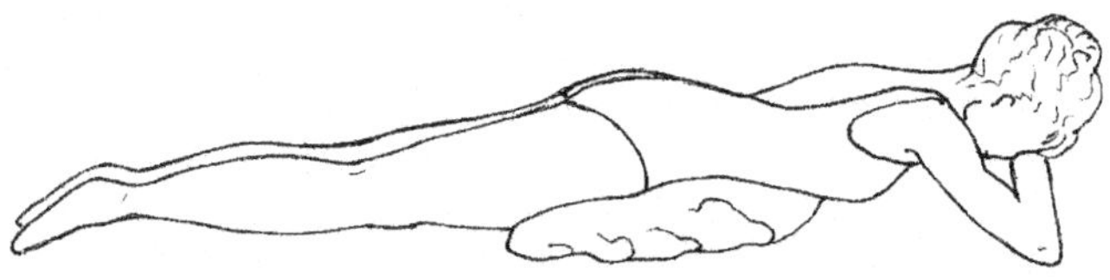

Starting Position

1. Start on your stomach, with or without a pillow under your belly (whichever is more comfortable).

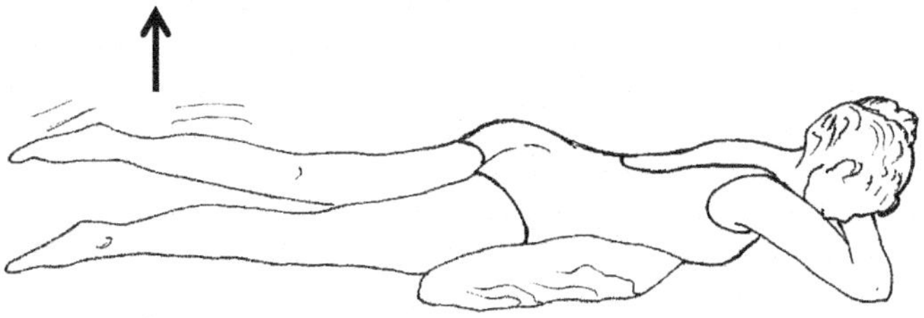

Exercise Movement

1. While keeping your leg *straight*, raise one leg up off the floor, hold it there for a second, then lower.
2. Do not arch your back or lift your leg up too high–around 6 inches or so is plenty.
3. Repeat with the other leg.
4. Do this over and over again, *alternating* the right and left legs, eventually working up to 20 repetitions over time *with each leg.*
5. Do this exercise one time a day, two to three days a week, with a day of rest in between.
6. When you can do this exercise for a total of 20 repetitions in a row with each leg, move on to Multifidus Strengthening Exercise #5.

Multifidus Strengthening Exercise #5 is the same exercise as #4 with the addition of ankle weights to increase the load on the multifidus and challenge it to become stronger. You'll likely need to start out with weights ranging anywhere from 1 to 5 pounds on each ankle. Once again, it's hard for me to tell you the exact amount of weight simply because I don't know how big or strong you are. Start out with a pound or two, and adjust as necessary so that you are able to do the exercise correctly *for at least 10 repetitions* or so.

Multifidus Strengthening Exercise #5

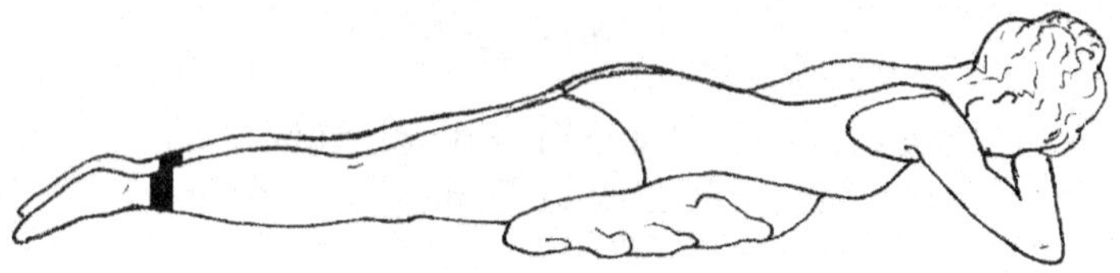

Starting Position

1. Lie on your stomach with your ankle weights on.
2. Place a pillow under your belly, if that's more comfortable.

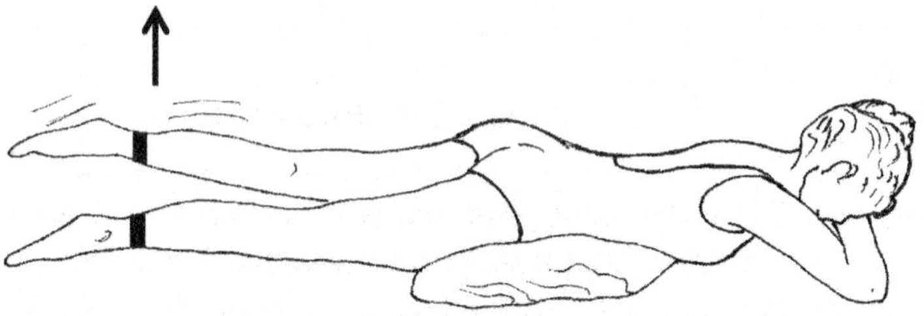

Exercise Movement

1. While keeping your leg *straight*, raise one leg up off the floor, hold it there for a second, then lower.
2. Do not arch your back or lift your leg up too high–around 6 inches or so is plenty.
3. Repeat with the other leg.
4. Do this over and over again, *alternating* the right and left legs, eventually working up to 20 repetitions over time *with each leg.*
5. Do this exercise one time a day, two to three days a week, with a day of rest in between.

a note on progressing and maintaining strength gains

When you've reached the point where you can do Exercise #5 for 20 repetitions (total of 20 times with the right leg and 20 times with the left leg) with light ankle weights, you are well on your way to building up good strength in your multifidus muscles. To continue to make them stronger, simply keep adding weight to the ankles progressively, a little at a time, until you feel that you're where you need to be, depending on your goals, job, activities, and such. Then, to maintain this strength, just do Multifidus Strengthening Exercise #5 once a week using the same weight, and doing the same amount of repetitions as you last did.

For example, let's say you feel that your back now has good strength and you can do Multifidus Strengthening Exercise #5 for 20 repetitions using 5-pound ankle weights on each leg. Doing Multifidus Strengthening Exercise #5 for 20 repetitions with the 5-pound ankle weights on each leg *once a week* is all that is necessary to keep current strength levels.

Okay. So far I have given you an exercise to be done on the hands and knees position, and one that can be done on the stomach. These two should cover the majority of readers. However, there still may be someone who can't get into any of these positions comfortably. Maybe you have knee trouble and can't get into the all fours position (or maybe you can but can't get out of it!). Or, maybe your back just talks to you too much while lying on your stomach. Whatever the case may be, this last exercise will work for you as long as you can either sit or stand.

This exercise is known as an *isometric* exercise, that is, an exercise where the muscle contracts but doesn't change its length. It may seem like a puny or trivial exercise, but this particular one has been shown in studies to actually *increase* the cross sectional area (or size) of the multifidus muscle (Hides 1996). And a multifidus that is bigger is definitely stronger!

Now this exercise is a bit tricky to do, so be sure to carefully follow all the instructions carefully. Here is the last multifidus strengthening exercise…

Multifidus Strengthening Exercise #6

1. Standing is preferable, but the exercise can be done while sitting as well.
2. Place one hand on your stomach muscles, and the other on your lower back multifidus muscles (see page 34 if you've forgotten how to find them).
3. The hands do nothing now, but will feel the muscles tighten later on in the exercise.

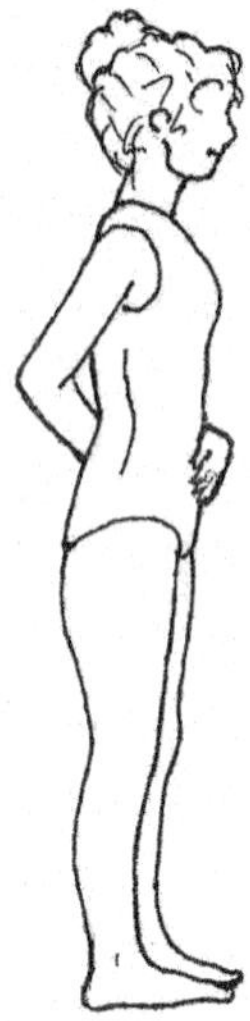

Starting Position

1. Tense up your stomach muscles by pulling your belly button *in and up* (see arrow in picture) while trying to keep your trunk and body still.
2. As you do this, *feel with your hands your stomach muscles and your lower back muscles tense and tighten up.*
3. Hold this position, muscles tightened, for a count of 3 to 5 seconds, and then relax your muscles.
4. Repeat, eventually working up to twenty repetitions in a row.
5. Make sure that when you tense the muscles, you try to do so as tightly as possible.
6. Do this exercise one time a day.
7. Good gains in strength can be made by doing this exercise at least three days a week with a day of rest in between.
8. Doing this exercise daily will bring even better strength gains.

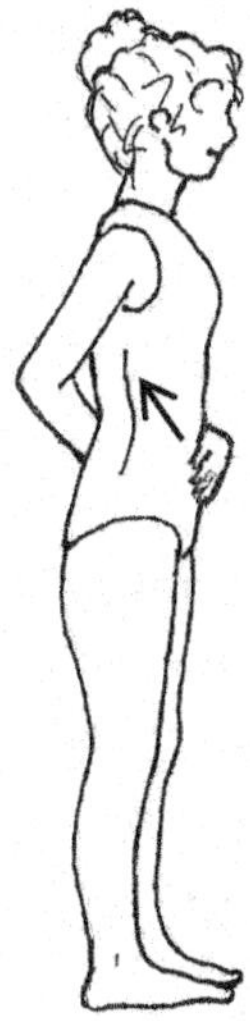

Exercise Movement

a note on progressing and maintaining strength gains

There is no way to add weight to this exercise in order to make it progressively harder on the multifidus. Rather, with the isometric exercise, *you* provide the stimulus to keep challenging the multifidus by always trying to tense the muscles as tightly as you comfortably can.

Continue doing 20 repetitions, holding each repetition for 3 to 5 seconds at least three times a week with a day of rest in between, or daily for even better strength gains, until you feel that you're where you need to be depending on your goal, job, activities, etc.

Then, to maintain this strength, just do Multifidus Strengthening Exercise #6 once a week. For example, doing just one set of 20 repetitions for 3 to 5 seconds once a week, while trying to tense the muscles as tightly as is comfortable, is all that is needed to keep current strength levels.

Summary

Alright, there you have it. One multifidus strengthening exercise you can do on your hands and knees, one on your stomach, and one that can be done in either sitting or standing. Don't worry about choosing one right now and trying it, because it will be later on towards the end of the book (Chapter 6) that I'll actually have you pick one, *and then we'll put it together with all the other exercises in the book for one simple weekly routine*. For now, the idea is to just get you familiar with the exercises.

But whichever one you *do* end up picking, be rest assured that many scientific studies show that your multifidus muscle is *highly* active and getting a good workout when you perform *any* of them (Ekstrom 2008, Stevens 2007, Ekstrom 2007, Arokoski 1999, Hides 1996). Oh yeah!

Quick Review

- ✓ **many studies point out that people with spinal stenosis have abnormalities in their back muscles, particularly with *the multifidus***
- ✓ **your back has many individual multifidus muscles that, when combined, run the entire length of your spine**
- ✓ **nerves that make the multifidus work come from just one segment of the spine, unlike other back muscles which get their nerves from several different segments, which helps to protect their function**
- ✓ **the multifidus attaches directly to the joints in your spine**
- ✓ **the multifidus can be easily felt in isolation in the *lower* back region**
- ✓ **a normal muscle is not painful to the touch–your multifidus shouldn't be either**
- ✓ **the multifidus is a highly active muscle in the back that is involved in *many* everyday motions and activities**
- ✓ **a back that has good stability can keep itself in safe positions and thereby avoid injury**
- ✓ **the muscles are a major source of stability for the spine–a human spine without muscles is unable to support normal loads**
- ✓ **the multifidus helps control the motions of the individual vertebrae**
- ✓ **when back muscles contract, they "stiffen" the spine, thereby stabilizing and protecting it**
- ✓ **about 2/3 of the total stiffness that the back muscles can produce for support through muscle contraction comes from the multifidus**
- ✓ **in order for muscles to continue to get stronger, they must be progressively challenged with more weight**
- ✓ **multiple randomized controlled trials point out that muscles can be adequately strengthened by doing just one set of an exercise to momentary muscular failure**
- ✓ **lower repetitions have a tendency to increase a muscle's *strength,* while higher repetitions (around 20 or more) have more of a tendency to increase a muscle's *endurance***
- ✓ **randomized controlled trials point out that strengthening exercises should be done two to three times a week in order to make a muscle stronger, and that once a week is enough to *preserve* strength gains**

4 Tune-Up #2: How to Make Your Back *More* Flexible

So far we've talked about restoring your back's muscular *strength.* While critically important, it's still only one piece of the puzzle when it comes to treating your spinal stenosis by improving the function of your spine. Why? Because the strongest back muscles in the world will do you little good if all you can do is move your spine back and forth a few degrees!

This brings us to the issue of back *flexibility*, or what physical therapists call *range on motion.* While it makes sense that a well-functioning spine should have good range of motion, I never add another exercise to a patient's already busy day unless I've got a good evidence-based reason to do so. Having said that, let's see what the research has to say about the back flexibility of people with spinal stenosis…

- one study took people with low back pain and compared their back range of motion to normal subjects (McGregor 1997)
- back pain patients were divided up into five different diagnostic groups. Some people had a herniated disc, some had degenerative disc disease, some had spondylolisthesis, some spinal stenosis, and others non-specific low back pain.
- of all the subjects in the study, those in the spinal stenosis group had the *worst* back flexibility

Apparently people with spinal stenosis have *really* poor spine flexibility–which is exactly what more recent studies have also discovered (Iversen 2009). No need to worry though, that's a problem we intent to tackle right now…

Use These Stretching Secrets to Succeed

While there are many different techniques to choose from when it comes to stretching out a tight muscle, by far the easiest and least complicated way is known as *the static stretch.* A static (or stationary) stretch takes a tight muscle, puts it in a lengthened position, and keeps it there for a certain period of time. For instance, if you wanted to use the static stretch technique to make the hamstring muscle on the back of your thigh more flexible, you could simply bend over with your knees straight and try to touch your toes. Thus, as you are holding this position, the muscle is being *statically stretched.* There's no bouncing, just a gentle, sustained stretch.

It sounds easy, perhaps a bit *too* easy, so you may be wondering at this point just how effective static stretching really is when it comes to making one more flexible. Well, a quick review of the stretching research pretty much lays it out straight as there are *multiple* randomized controlled trials clearly in agreement that this is a winning method. Here are the highlights…

- a study published in the journal *Physical Therapy* took 57 subjects and randomly divided them up into four groups (Bandy 1994).
- the first group held their static stretch for a length of 15 seconds, the second group for 30 seconds, and the third for 60. The fourth group (the control group) did not stretch at all.
- all three groups performed *one* stretch a day, five days a week, for six weeks
- results showed that holding a stretch for a period of 30 seconds was just as effective at increasing flexibility as holding one for 60 seconds. Also, holding a stretch for a period of 30 seconds was much more effective than holding one for 15 seconds or (of course) not stretching at all.

Hmm. Looks like if you hold a stretch for 15 seconds, it doesn't do much to make you more flexible. On the other hand, holding a stretch for 30 full seconds *does* work–and just as well as 60 seconds.

Wow. So now that we know 30 seconds seems to be the magic number, makes you wonder if doing *a bunch* of 30-second stretches would be *even better* than doing it one time like they did in the study...

- another randomized controlled trial done several years later (Bandy 1997) set out to research not only the optimal length of time to hold a static stretch, *but also the optimal number of times to do it*
- 93 subjects were recruited and randomly placed into one of five groups: 1) perform three 1-minute stretches; 2) perform three 30-second stretches; 3) perform a 1-minute stretch; 4) perform a 30-second stretch; or 5) do no stretching at all (the control group)
- the results? Not so surprising was the fact that all groups that stretched became more flexible than the control group that didn't stretch.
- however what *was* surprising was the finding that among the groups that did stretch, no one group became more flexible than the other!
- in other words, the researchers found that as far as trying to become more flexible, it made no difference whether the stretching time was increased from 30 to 60 seconds, OR when the frequency was changed from doing one stretch a day to doing three stretches a day

So here we have yet *another* randomized controlled trial (the kind of study that provides the highest form of proof in medicine) which is showing us once again that holding a stretch for 30-seconds is *just as effective* as holding it for 60 seconds. And to top it all off, doing the 30-second stretch *once* is just as good as if you did it three times!

Interestingly, other randomized controlled trials have also supported the effectiveness of the 30-second stretch done one time a day, five days a week, to make one more flexible (Bandy 1998). Fantastic!

So as the randomized controlled trials *clearly* point out, it really doesn't take a lot of time to stretch out tight muscles *if* you know how. Based on the current published stretching research, this book recommends the following guidelines for the average person needing to stretch out a tight muscle with the static stretch technique:

- get into the starting position
- next, begin moving into the stretch position until a *gentle* stretch is felt
- once this position is achieved, hold for a full 30 seconds
- when the 30 seconds is up, *slowly* release the stretch
- do this one time a day, five days a week

One last note. While it is acceptable to feel a little discomfort while doing a stretch, it is *not* okay to be in pain. Do not force yourself to get into any stretching position, and by all means, skip the stretch entirely if it makes your pain worse.

It Only Takes *Three* Stretches to Get the Job Done

Okay, time for the meat and potatoes of the chapter–the stretches! While there are a ton of stretches I *could* have you do, I'm only going to give you *three*. Why only three? Well, while your spine can move in a bunch of different ways, if you break it down, there are really only four basic motions. They are:

- *flexion*, which is bending forward
- *extension*, which is bending backwards
- *rotation*, which is twisting to the right or left
- *sidebending*, which is leaning to the left or right

So the stretches in this book will be designed to improve 3 of the 4 basic motions of your back: flexion, rotation, and sidebending. Why not extension? Because when you extend your back, or lean backwards, this motion actually makes the already narrowed "holes" in your back where the nerves come out *even smaller*–a motion that people with spinal stenosis want to avoid doing a lot of.

Back Stretch #1: Increase Flexion

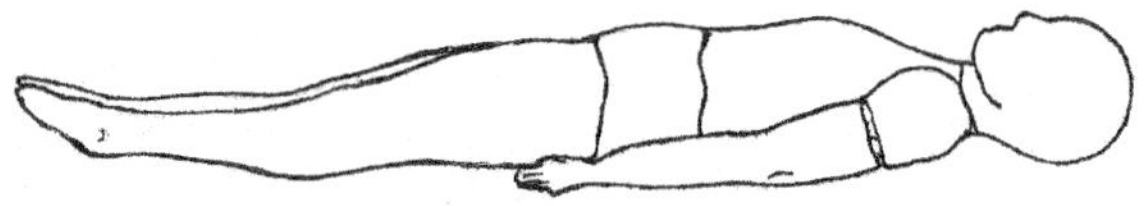

1. Get into the same position as the above picture.
2. You should be lying on your back–place a pillow under your head if necessary.

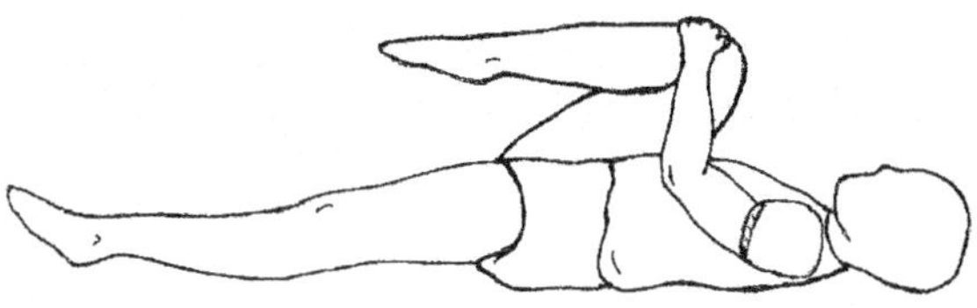

1. Using both hands, smoothly pull one of your knees straight up towards your chest until you feel a gentle stretch in your low back/hip area.
2. Hold for a full 30 seconds, then gently release the leg back to the floor.
3. Repeat with the other leg.

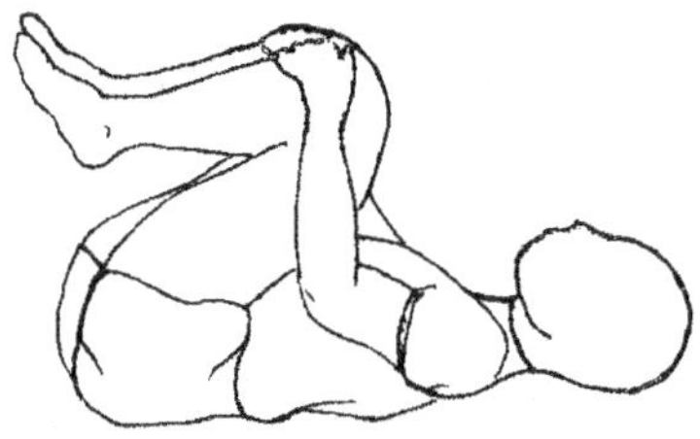

1. For a stronger stretch, you can smoothly pull *both* knees straight up towards your chest (at the same time) until you feel a gentle stretch in your low back/hip area.
2. Hold for a full 30 seconds, then gently release both legs back to the floor.

Back Stretch #2: Increase Rotation

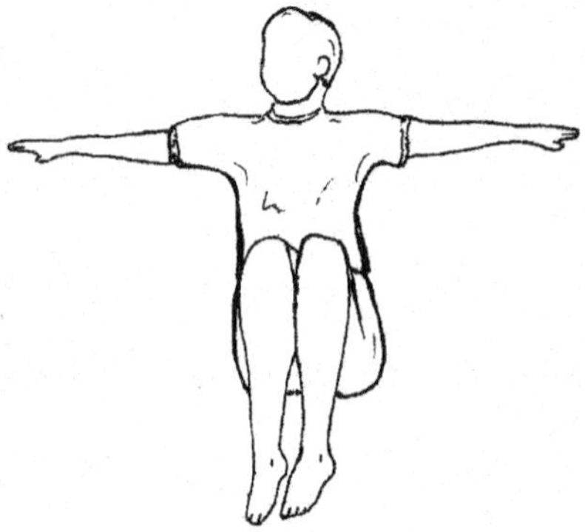

1. Get into the same position as the above picture.
2. You should be lying on your back with both knees bent comfortably. Both feet should also be flat on the floor.
3. It is preferable to keep you arms in the same position as the picture, but you can lower them a bit if it is more comfortable.

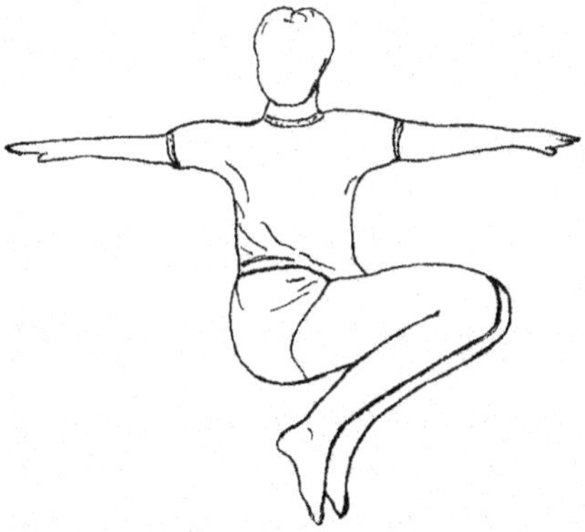

1. *Keeping your shoulders and arms in place and on the floor*, flop your knees over to one side until you feel a gentle stretch in your low back/hip area. You should be in the same position as the above picture.
2. Hold for a full 30 seconds, then gently return to the starting position.
3. Next, repeat this same motion, *going to the other side*.

Back Stretch #3: Increase Sidebending

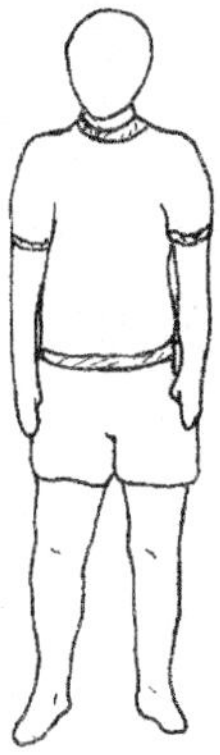

1. Get into the same position as the above picture.
2. You should be standing up straight with your arms at your side, feet comfortably apart.

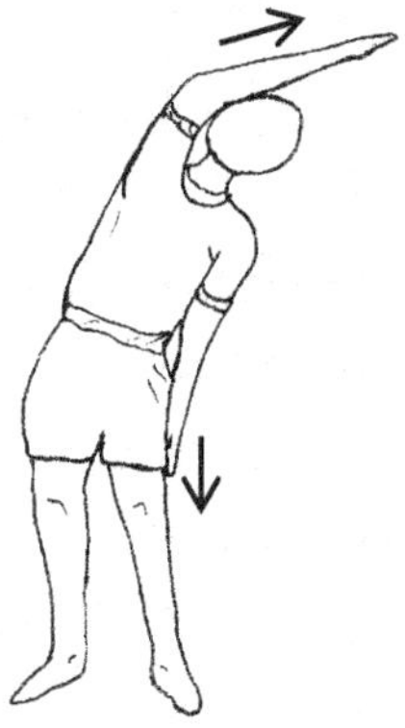

1. Keeping your feet in place, lift one arm up over your head, *while leaning to the side* as in the above picture. The other arm slides *down* your side.
2. Continue leaning over until you feel a gentle stretching of your side and lower back.
3. Hold for a full 30 seconds, then gently return to the starting position.
4. Repeat this same motion *going to the other side.*
5. Note: If raising your arm over your head is really uncomfortable, you can skip it and just concentrate more on the arm that is sliding down your side.

Not too bad, huh? By using these evidence-based stretching techniques, you will be sending a clear signal to your muscles that they need to elongate and stretch out.

Then, over a period of weeks, the tissues will begin to gradually lengthen, bit by bit–which means *more* flexibility for your back. Know too that these stretches also help loosen up other tight spinal structures as well, such as the tiny facet joints.

Quick Review

- ✓ **many studies have found that patients with spinal stenosis have decreased back flexibility**
- ✓ **one of the easiest and most effective ways of becoming more flexible is to use the *static stretching* technique**
- ✓ **according to randomized controlled trials, holding a static stretch for 15 seconds does little to increase one's flexibility. On the other hand, holding a static stretch for 30 seconds is just as effective as holding one for 60 seconds.**
- ✓ **randomized controlled trials point out that doing one 30-second static stretch is just as effective as doing *three* 30-second static stretches**
- ✓ **randomized controlled trials also point out that doing your static stretching exercises five times a week is quite sufficient to make your muscles longer**

5 Tune-Up #3: How to Improve Your *Proprioception*

While the word proprioception may look confusing, all this fourteen-letter word means is the ability you have at any given moment to sense the position and movements of your body. For example, if you close your eyes, you could probably tell me without difficulty if your knees are bent or straight, or if your head is turned to the left or right–all without even looking. To give you more of an idea of just how useful proprioception is, here are a few everyday activities whose success or failure depends on the proper functioning of your sense of proprioception…

- getting keys out of your pocket
- pushing down on the gas or brake pedal in your car
- walking in the dark to the bathroom
- scratching that hard-to-reach spot on your back

As you can see, all of these particular activities involve getting something done without the help of your vision. By giving your brain constant updates as to the position of your body parts, your proprioception helps you out a lot when you are unable to see exactly what you are doing.

Another good example of how crucial this sense of proprioception is to our day-to-day existence comes from a patient I had once who lacked proprioception in both his legs. Unfortunately, this gentleman suffered from a condition called CIDP, or *chronic inflammatory demyelinating polyneruropathy*, a rare neurological disorder involving destruction of the covering around the nerves. As his physical therapist, it was my job was to get him out of the bed and see how well he could walk.

The first hurdle we had to cross, getting him on his feet, proved to be somewhat easy–we used a walker and his legs were quite strong. Walking, however, turned out to be another matter entirely, as each step was like a journey into the unknown. Since his legs gave him little feedback as to where they actually were, his whole leg would begin to swing wildly in a circular motion, as he desperately tried to place his foot accurately on the floor. Even though he *knew* where he wanted his legs to go, and had plenty of strength to make them move, it was impractical for him to walk any meaningful distance without good proprioception.

Now it needs to be said that having proprioception problems to this degree usually occurs when one has a *serious* problem with his or her nervous system. Perhaps that's why proprioception exercises are usually *last* on the list of treatments when it comes to problems such as back pain–a lot of medical professionals simply tend to think of proprioception problems as only happening in patients with grave neurological disorders. However this is clearly *not* the case. It took some time, but back researchers are now getting around to checking out the proprioception in the low backs of people with spinal stenosis–and guess what they're finding...

- researchers took 26 patients with spinal stenosis and tested the proprioception in their lumbar spine (Leinonen 2002)
- to do this, subjects were placed in a seated position while the seat was slowly rotated. The subject then indicated the movement by releasing a finger switch. Also, subjects were asked to localize the area of sensation, as well as the direction of movement.
- results revealed that 20 out of 26 patients reported the movement direction *incorrectly*
- furthermore, patients consistently localized the movement sensation in their shoulders, instead of their low back

This study clearly shows us that *many* people with spinal stenosis have much difficulty sensing rotational movements in their low backs–indicating a problem with proprioception And so, this next exercise is designed to specifically challenge your spinal proprioception and tune-up it up...

Spinal Proprioception Exercise

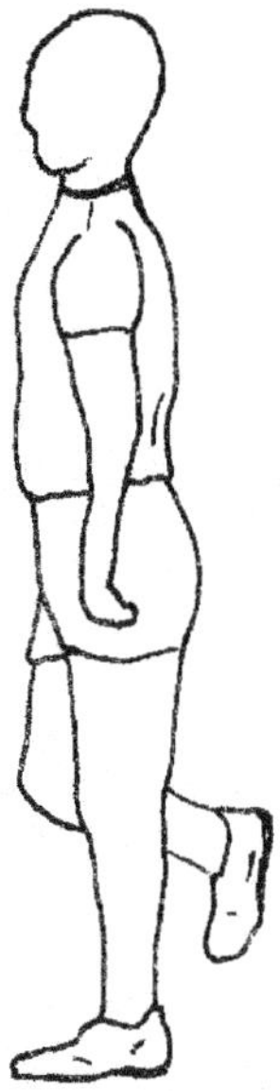

1. Stand on one leg in the same position as the above picture. Your knee can be straight or slightly bent, whichever is more comfortable.
2. If you can't balance well on one leg at all, or if you feel like you might fall, stand next to a table, chair, or doorway–something you can lightly hold on to.
3. Try to stay standing on one leg for 30 full seconds.
4. When you can stand on one leg, well-balanced, for 30 full seconds *without holding on to anything*, it's time to make it more challenging by closing your eyes.
5. When you can stand on one leg, well balanced, for 30 full seconds, without holding on to anything *and your eyes closed,* you can try for 60 seconds for an advanced challenge.
6. If you find you simply cannot stand on one leg without holding on to something, that's okay, just follow the same progression above, except hold on as lightly as you safely can.

A few comments about this exercise. Number one, it's much harder than it looks. If at first glance you're thinking, "That looks too easy" –give it a try. If you can stand on one leg, well balanced, for 60 full seconds with your eyes closed, you can skip it as far as I'm concerned.

And how often do you need to do it? Well, since there's little research telling us how often a person needs to do this exercise to get *the best* results, I recommend doing it three times a week with a day of rest in between, just as with the multifidus strengthening exercise. Week-by-week, the exercise will begin to get easier and easier, indicating that you're well on your way to improving your proprioception.

The other thing, is that this exercise may not seem like it's much of an exercise that involves your back–but it is. Watching many patients over the years trying to do this exercise, I usually see their trunks moving around quite a bit as they struggle to hold the one-leg position–a good indication that their spinal joint and muscle proprioceptors are being stimulated. The research has also confirmed that standing balance activities cause much EMG activity of the back muscles (Burton 1986) –which means they're getting a work out!

Quick Review

- ✓ **proprioception is your ability to sense the position and movements of your body**
- ✓ **studies show that many people with spinal stenosis have abnormal proprioception in their low back**
- ✓ **standing balance activities are one good way to challenge your back proprioceptors**

6 Putting It All Together: The Six-Week Program

The first exercise program I ever wrote for publication consisted of three exercises, and I asked the reader to choose *only one.* The exercises were shown to be effective in randomized controlled trials, and if the diligent reader truly followed my specific, evidence-based guidelines, I could all but guarantee that their pain would improve, if not go away altogether.

Eventually the book was translated into other languages, and as its popularity grew, I started getting some interesting feedback from worldwide readers. Two points consistently came up regarding this exercise routine:

- there weren't enough exercises in the book
- the exercises were too simple *or* they were ones that readers had already seen/done before

In case some of these same issues bother you as you review the exercise routine in this chapter, I would like to take a moment out to dispel a few common misconceptions. The first one is that some people think you have to spend *a lot* of time doing *a lot* of exercises in order to get better–which is simply untrue.

If your exercise program truly targets the *correct* problems with *effective* exercises, then you should not be spending all day doing dozens of exercises. Of course there are exceptions, but they are few.

Another misconception is that simple, uncomplicated exercises are ineffective. Take stretching for example. Pulling one knee up towards your chest, and holding it there for a mere thirty-seconds, once a day, may appear to some readers to be too simple a maneuver or too short a time frame to ever stretch out tight muscles. But on the contrary, multiple randomized controlled trials have *consistently* pointed out that stretching for a longer period of time, or more times a day, will *not* produce better results.

And finally, the last common misconception deals with not trying an exercise because, "I've done that one before and it didn't help." The interesting thing I've noted, is that when you question someone carefully about what they actually did, you often find that while a person may in fact have been doing an exercise correctly, they have *not* been following proper evidence-based guidelines. Using stretching as an example again, let's say that a person tries a particular stretch that is indeed targeting the correct tight muscle, only they've been holding the stretch for *fifteen-seconds* instead of the proven *thirty-seconds.*

After getting poor results for a period of time, most people will usually abandon the exercise and think, "That stretch didn't work." The truth, however, is that they really were doing a helpful exercise, it's just that they weren't following the correct evidence-based guidelines to make the exercise effective.

The moral? When proceeding with the exercises in this book, make sure that you do them *exactly* as instructed, even if you've tried some of them before or they seem too simple to be effective. Then and only then can you say with certainty that the exercises in this book were really helpful or not.

So, with that out of the way, I'm now going to answer a few questions most patients usually ask when I go over an exercise routine with them. After that, we'll move right into the six-week program. Okay, first question…

What should I wear?

Nothing fancy. You'll want to wear something loose that allows you to move your arms and legs around freely. The last thing you really want is to wear is a tight shirt that keeps you from lifting your arms up, or a pair of jeans that keeps you from bending your knees. Also, try not to wear clothing that will cause you to overheat and get hot while exercising–which of course will vary from person to person.

What equipment will I need?

Since you'll be doing a strengthening exercise that involves lifting weights, it's a no-brainer that you'll at least need some kind of weight to pick up and move around. But, does this mean that all you'll need is a can of beans or a dumbbell? Well, you'll need a little more than that. Remember from our discussion on page 39 that muscles get stronger only when we constantly challenge them to do more than they're used to doing. So, this means that taking the same weight, and lifting it over and over again, week after week, simply won't get the job done. Therefore, you'll need to have *several* weights of varying pounds available to use.

Now if you think this will involve a lot of money, it doesn't have to. By far, the easiest and cheapest way to go is to buy a set of *adjustable* ankle weights. You can get them at most sporting good stores and they typically look something like this:

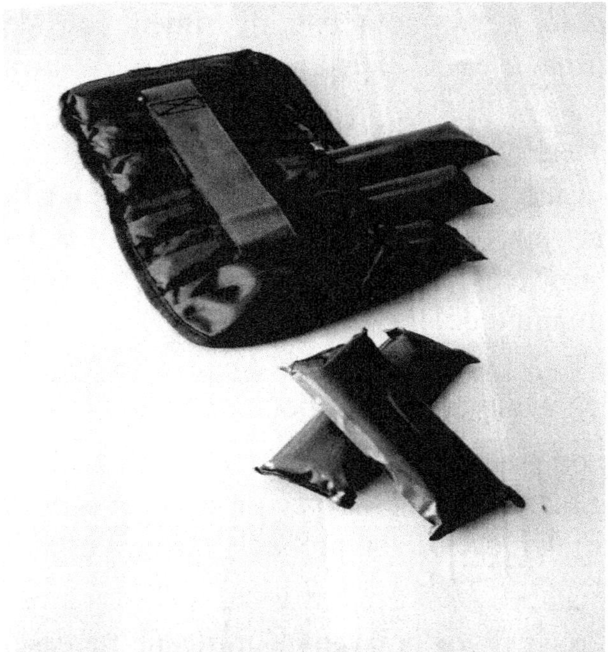

As you can see from the picture, the cuff can attach quite easily to your ankle or wrist by means of a velcro strap. Also note that the cuff is made up of six mini weight packs that you can take in and out of their little pockets, depending on how many pounds you want to use. Since the cuff in the picture weighs a total of 10 pounds, and has six little packs, this means that each one weighs a little over a pound and a half. This allows you to increase the weight *gradually* on any given exercise–which is one of the biggest advantages of using *adjustable* cuff weights.

Some tips on buying them. First, be aware that there are *wrist* cuffs and there are *ankle* cuffs (the above picture shows an ankle cuff). Wrist cuffs are smaller, but I recommend getting the ankle cuffs, mainly because they are heavier which allows you to go up higher in weight over time than the wrist cuffs. Second, pay particular attention to how many total pounds *each cuff* weighs. How much weight should you look for? Probably two 10-pound cuffs will give you a good workout for awhile. If the need arises, they do make two 20-pound cuffs which are also widely available.

As far as cost, I have priced these cuffs at a lot of places and the average cost is around twenty dollars for a pair–not a bad investment considering one pair should last for years with normal use.

The Six-Week Program

Up to this point in the book, we've built a good foundation of knowledge for you to be able to treat your own spinal stenosis. With that accomplished, it's now time to go over the six-week program I've laid out for you. Here are a few key rules to always keep in mind before you begin …

- always check with your doctor before beginning an exercise program
- the number one rule is "Do no harm." You should not be in a lot of pain while doing these exercises. Some discomfort is okay, but remember that you're working muscles you probably haven't used in a while, at least in this manner.
- stop the exercise if you have any significant increase in back pain or symptoms. If done correctly, the exercises in this book do not stretch your back in odd or unsafe positions, nor do they involve any heavy weights–and should be safe for your back. *However*, it's your back and your responsibility to stop if you feel like any harm is being done.

So does this home exercise program *really* work? Well, as we've said before, the best way in medicine to prove that something works is to conduct a randomized controlled trial–as this type of study provides the highest proof possible that a treatment is really effective. Here's an example of one that involved spinal stenosis patients…

- 29 patients with spinal stenosis were randomly assigned to one of three groups (Koc 2009)
- one group received inpatient physical therapy, a home exercise program, and pain medications
- another group got epidural steroid injections, a home exercise program, and pain medications
- the control group *only* got a home exercise program consisting of stretching and strengthening exercises and pain medications
- all groups showed significant improvements throughout the study, *including the control group*

As you can see, it's quite possible for spinal stenosis patients to improve symptoms on their own, with a simple home program, consisting of stretching and strengthening exercises. Having said that, here's the six-week program designed to treat your spinal stenosis by improving the functioning of your back…

DO THESE EXERCISES ON MONDAY, WEDNESDAY, and FRIDAY

Increases Back Flexibility			Increases Back Strength	Increases Back Proprioception
Back Stretch #1: Increase Flexion	**Back Stretch #2: Increase Rotation**	**Back Stretch #3: Increase Sidebending**	**Multifidus Strengthening Exercise (Pick One)**	**Spinal Proprioception Exercise**
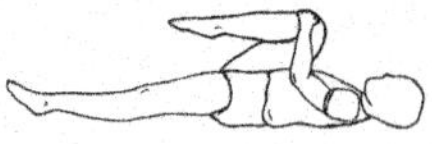	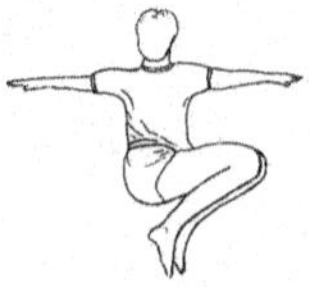	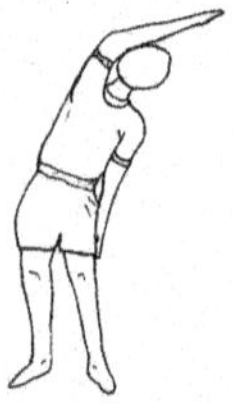	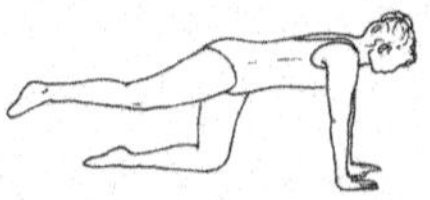 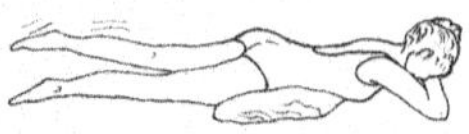 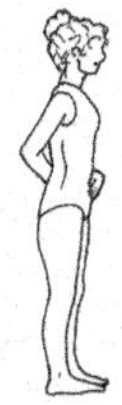	
hold for 30 sec. x 1 each leg	hold for 30 sec. x 1 each side	hold for 30 sec. x 1 each side	1 set x 10-20 reps	start out trying for 30 seconds
p. 61	p. 62	p. 63	pgs. 47-54	p. 67

DO THESE EXERCISES ON TUESDAY and THURSDAY

Increases Back Flexibility		
Back Stretch #1: Increase Flexion	**Back Stretch #2: Increase Rotation**	**Back Stretch #3: Increase Sidebending**
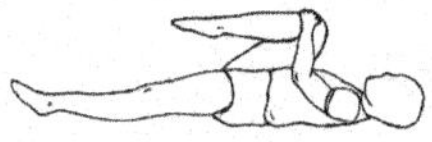	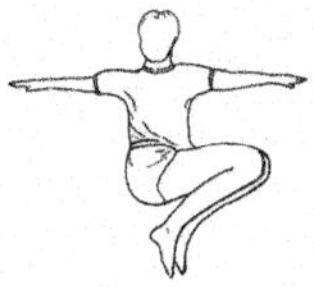	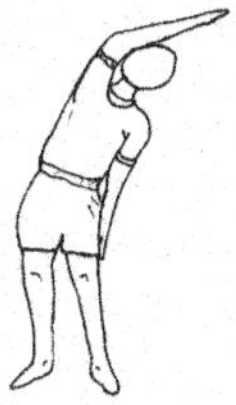 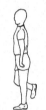
hold for 30 sec. x 1 each leg	hold for 30 sec. x 1 each side	hold for 30 sec. x 1 each side
p. 61	p. 62	p. 63

Track Your Progress!

Since it can be hard to remember from one session to the next what weight you used or how many seconds you stood on one leg, it's helpful to quickly jot down this information. I've also found that when patients keep track of their exercises, it helps keep them on track too! The following is an example of how to record your progress by using the exercise sheets provided in this book…

Week 3: Exercise Session #4
Thursday

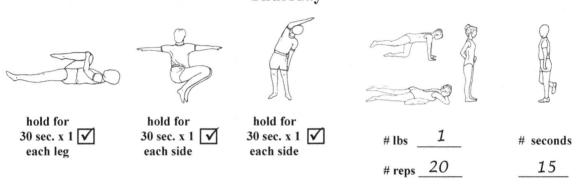

hold for 30 sec. x 1 ☑ each leg	hold for 30 sec. x 1 ☑ each side	hold for 30 sec. x 1 ☑ each side	# lbs 1 # reps 20	# seconds 15

Using the exercise sheets provided is easy. *Looking left to right,* you just have to put a check in the box *after* you do each of the stretches.

Next, you'll see that there are three pictures of the multifidus strengthening exercises–which *doesn't* mean you do them all. Rather, they're all pictured because not everyone will be doing the same one. As you can see, this person used a one-pound ankle weight on each leg, and so they simply wrote a "1" down in the space provided. Also note that they were able to do 20 reps, so they should *increase* the weight by a pound or so next session. And finally, since they could stand on one leg for 15 seconds, they simply jotted down a "15" under the picture of that exercise. Next time, maybe they can stand on one leg for 20 or 25 seconds.

The pages that follow contain exercise sheets for six weeks of workouts. Make additional copies as needed. And don't miss the ***Quickstart Guide*** that is included at the end of this chapter to get you started.

Week 1: Exercise Session #1
Monday

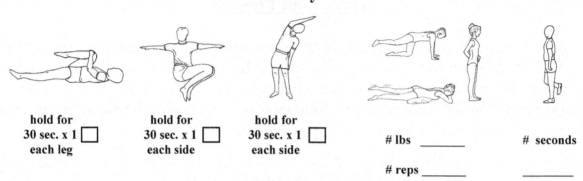

hold for
30 sec. x 1 ☐
each leg

hold for
30 sec. x 1 ☐
each side

hold for
30 sec. x 1 ☐
each side

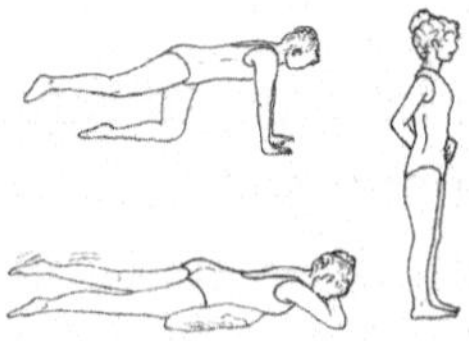

lbs _______

reps _______

seconds

____

Week 1: Exercise Session #2
Tuesday

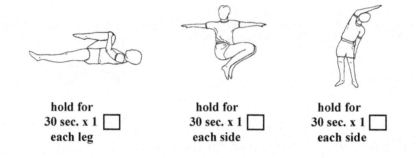

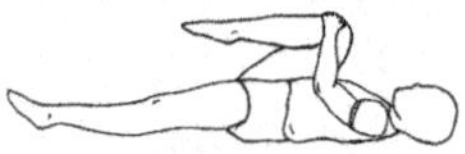

hold for
30 sec. x 1 ☐
each leg

hold for
30 sec. x 1 ☐
each side

hold for
30 sec. x 1 ☐
each side

Week 1: Exercise Session #3
Wednesday

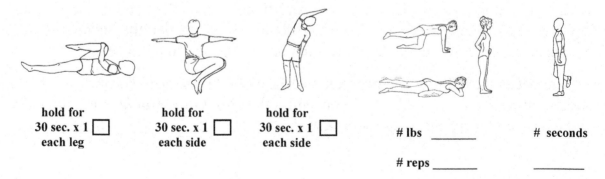

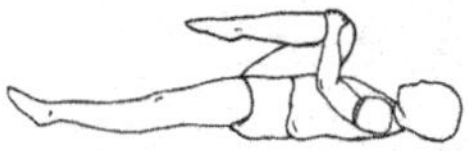

hold for
30 sec. x 1 ☐
each leg

hold for
30 sec. x 1 ☐
each side

hold for
30 sec. x 1 ☐
each side

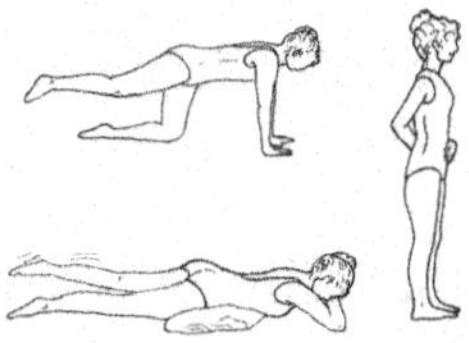

lbs _______

reps _______

seconds

____

Week 1: Exercise Session #4
Thursday

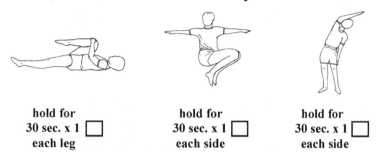

hold for
30 sec. x 1 ☐
each leg

hold for
30 sec. x 1 ☐
each side

hold for
30 sec. x 1 ☐
each side

Week 1: Exercise Session #5
Friday

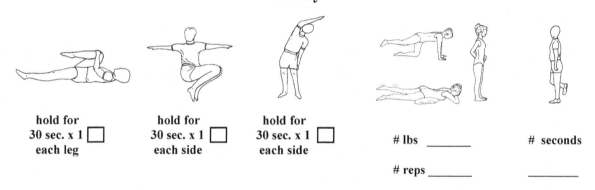

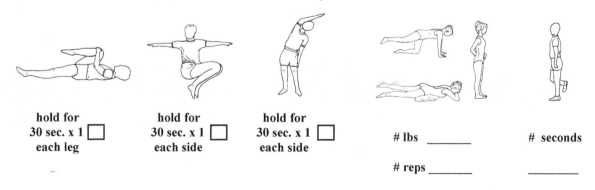

hold for
30 sec. x 1 ☐
each leg

hold for
30 sec. x 1 ☐
each side

hold for
30 sec. x 1 ☐
each side

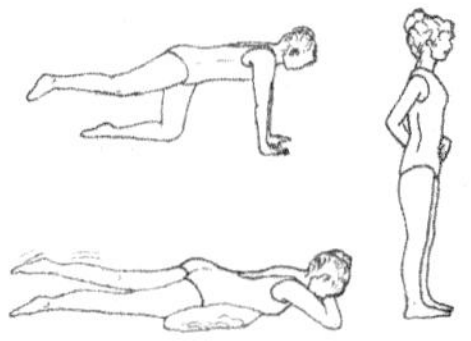

lbs _______

reps _______

seconds

____

Week 2: Exercise Session #1
Monday

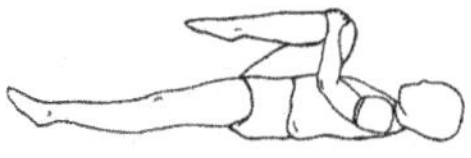

hold for
30 sec. x 1 ☐
each leg

hold for
30 sec. x 1 ☐
each side

hold for
30 sec. x 1 ☐
each side

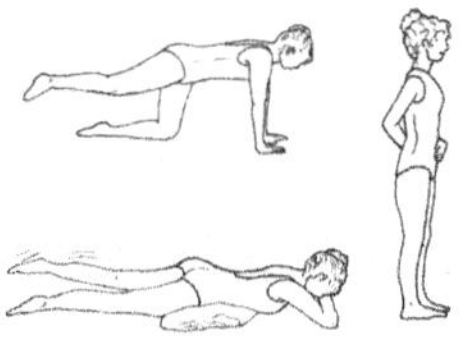

lbs _______

reps _______

seconds

____

Week 2: Exercise Session #2
Tuesday

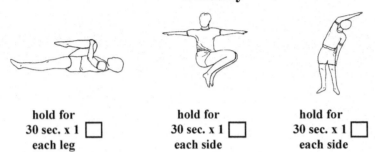

hold for
30 sec. x 1 ☐
each leg

hold for
30 sec. x 1 ☐
each side

hold for
30 sec. x 1 ☐
each side

Week 2: Exercise Session #3
Wednesday

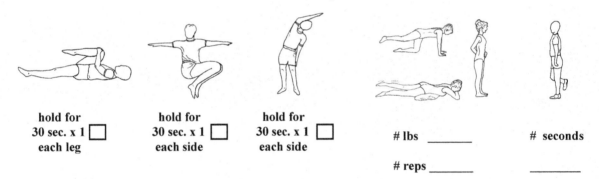

hold for
30 sec. x 1 ☐
each leg

hold for
30 sec. x 1 ☐
each side

hold for
30 sec. x 1 ☐
each side

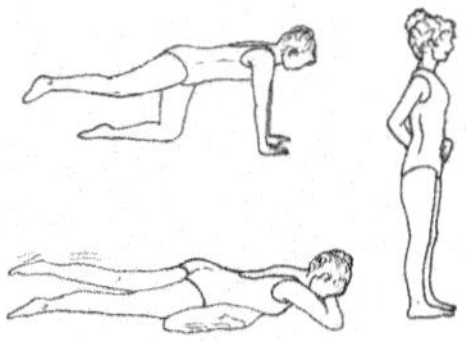

lbs _______

reps _______

seconds

____

Week 2: Exercise Session #4
Thursday

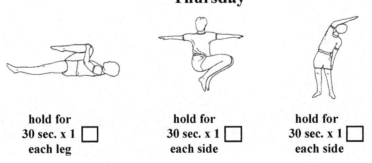

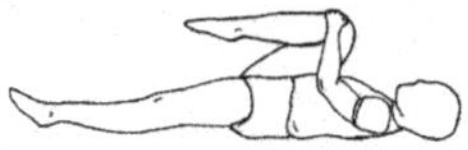

hold for
30 sec. x 1 ☐
each leg

hold for
30 sec. x 1 ☐
each side

hold for
30 sec. x 1 ☐
each side

Week 2: Exercise Session #5
Friday

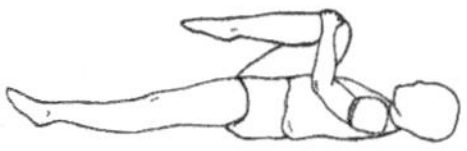

hold for
30 sec. x 1 ☐
each leg

hold for
30 sec. x 1 ☐
each side

hold for
30 sec. x 1 ☐
each side

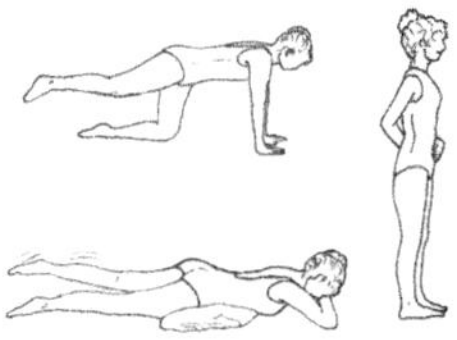

lbs _______

reps _______

seconds

____

Week 3: Exercise Session #1
Monday

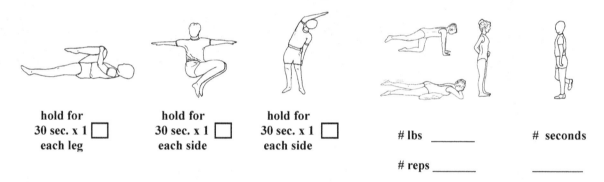

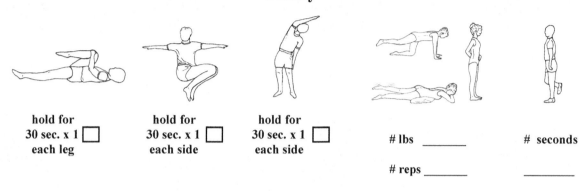

hold for
30 sec. x 1 ☐
each leg

hold for
30 sec. x 1 ☐
each side

hold for
30 sec. x 1 ☐
each side

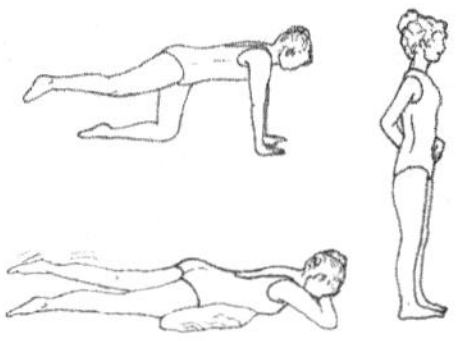

lbs _______

reps _______

seconds

____

Week 3: Exercise Session #2
Tuesday

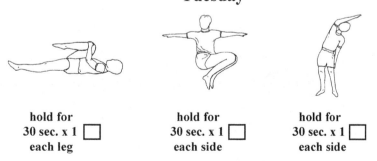

hold for
30 sec. x 1 ☐
each leg

hold for
30 sec. x 1 ☐
each side

hold for
30 sec. x 1 ☐
each side

Week 3: Exercise Session #3
Wednesday

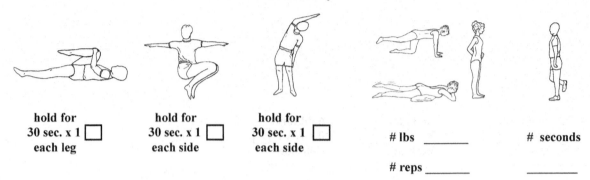

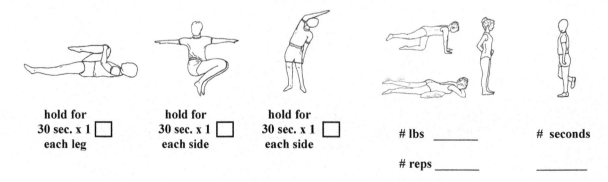

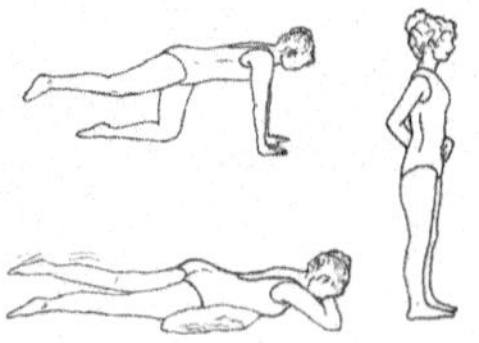

hold for
30 sec. x 1 ☐
each leg

hold for
30 sec. x 1 ☐
each side

hold for
30 sec. x 1 ☐
each side

lbs _______

reps _______

seconds

____

Week 3: Exercise Session #4
Thursday

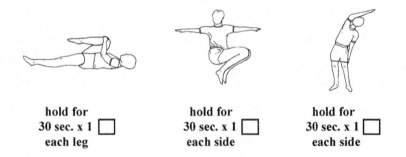

hold for
30 sec. x 1 ☐
each leg

hold for
30 sec. x 1 ☐
each side

hold for
30 sec. x 1 ☐
each side

Week 3: Exercise Session #5
Friday

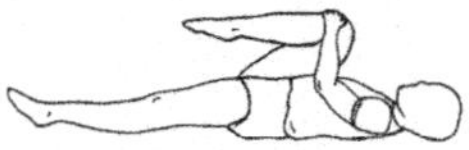

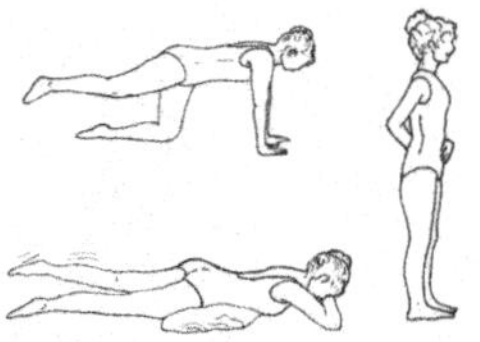

hold for
30 sec. x 1 ☐
each leg

hold for
30 sec. x 1 ☐
each side

hold for
30 sec. x 1 ☐
each side

lbs _______

reps _______

seconds

____

Week 4: Exercise Session #1
Monday

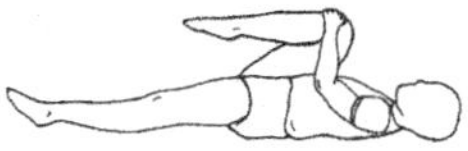

hold for
30 sec. x 1 ☐
each leg

hold for
30 sec. x 1 ☐
each side

hold for
30 sec. x 1 ☐
each side

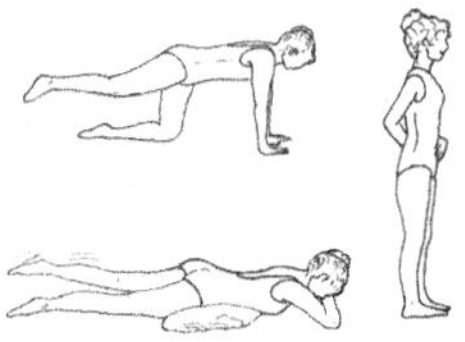

lbs _______

reps _______

seconds

____

Week 4: Exercise Session #2
Tuesday

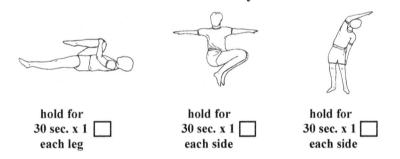

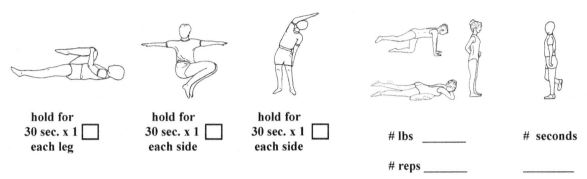

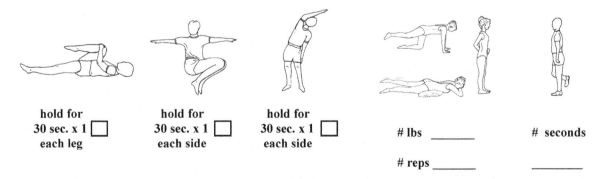

hold for
30 sec. x 1 ☐
each leg

hold for
30 sec. x 1 ☐
each side

hold for
30 sec. x 1 ☐
each side

Week 4: Exercise Session #3
Wednesday

hold for
30 sec. x 1 ☐
each leg

hold for
30 sec. x 1 ☐
each side

hold for
30 sec. x 1 ☐
each side

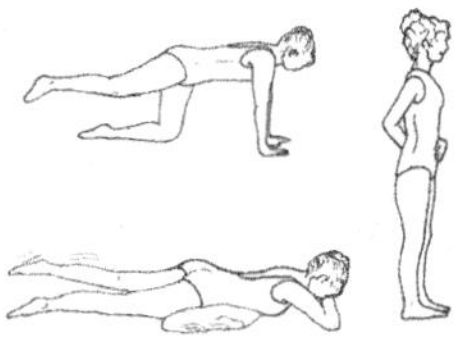

lbs _______

reps _______

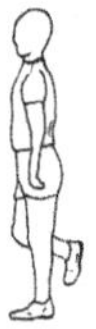

seconds

____

Week 4: Exercise Session #4
Thursday

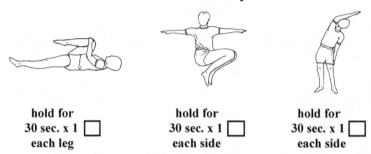

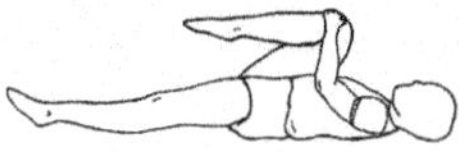

hold for
30 sec. x 1 ☐
each leg

hold for
30 sec. x 1 ☐
each side

hold for
30 sec. x 1 ☐
each side

Week 4: Exercise Session #5
Friday

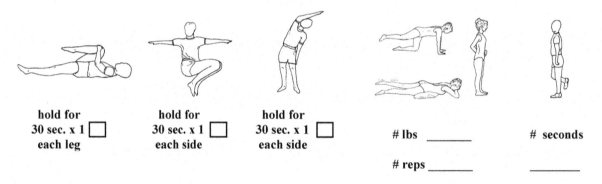

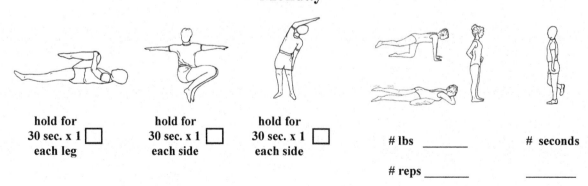

hold for
30 sec. x 1 ☐
each leg

hold for
30 sec. x 1 ☐
each side

hold for
30 sec. x 1 ☐
each side

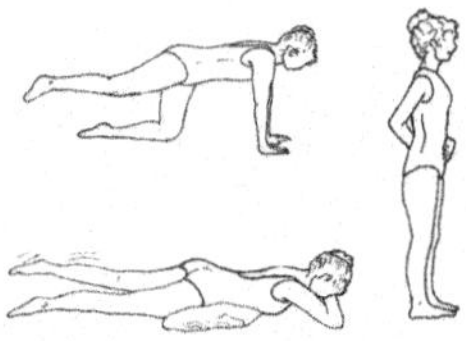

lbs _______

reps _______

seconds

____

Week 5: Exercise Session #1
Monday

hold for
30 sec. x 1 ☐
each leg

hold for
30 sec. x 1 ☐
each side

hold for
30 sec. x 1 ☐
each side

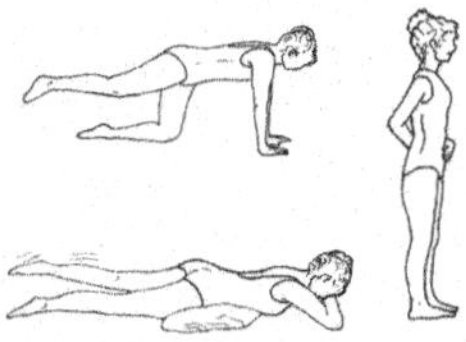

lbs _______

reps _______

seconds

____

Week 5: Exercise Session #2
Tuesday

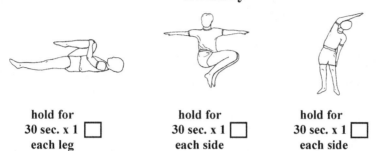

hold for
30 sec. x 1 ☐
each leg

hold for
30 sec. x 1 ☐
each side

hold for
30 sec. x 1 ☐
each side

Week 5: Exercise Session #3
Wednesday

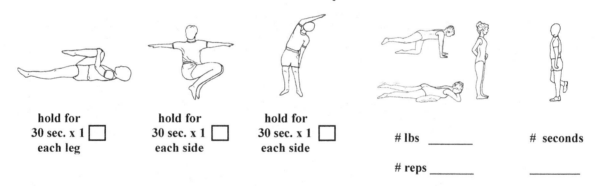

hold for
30 sec. x 1 ☐
each leg

hold for
30 sec. x 1 ☐
each side

hold for
30 sec. x 1 ☐
each side

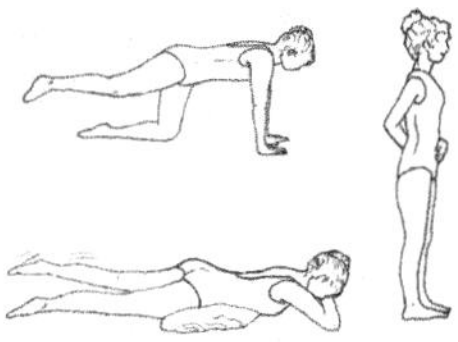

lbs _______

reps _______

seconds

____

Week 5: Exercise Session #4
Thursday

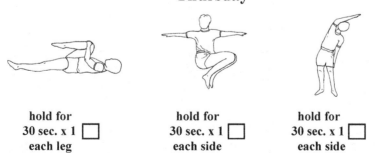

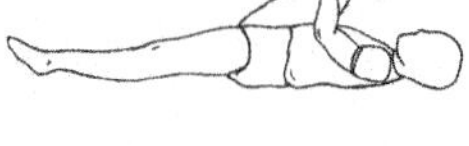

hold for
30 sec. x 1 ☐
each leg

hold for
30 sec. x 1 ☐
each side

hold for
30 sec. x 1 ☐
each side

Week 5: Exercise Session #5
Friday

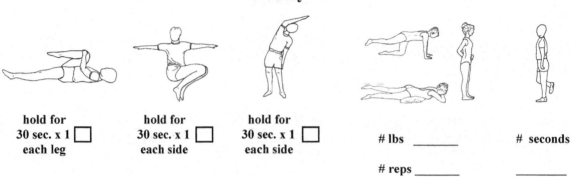

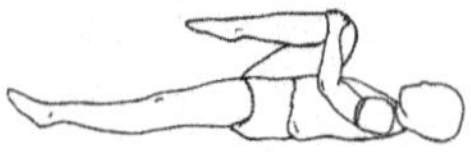

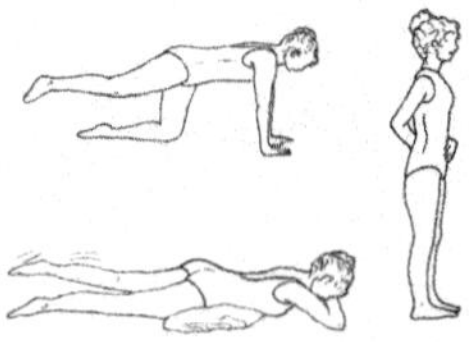

hold for 30 sec. x 1 ☐ each leg	hold for 30 sec. x 1 ☐ each side	hold for 30 sec. x 1 ☐ each side	# lbs _______ # reps _______	# seconds ________

Week 6: Exercise Session #1
Monday

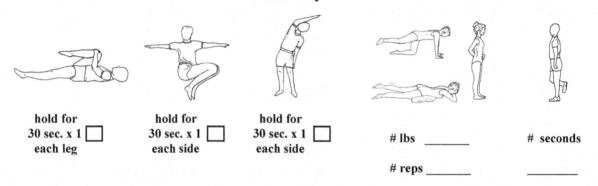

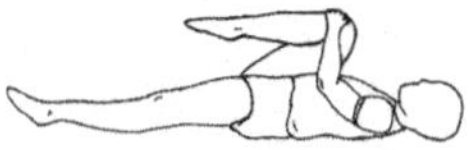

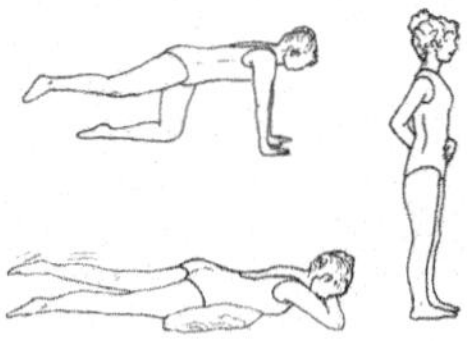

hold for 30 sec. x 1 ☐ each leg	hold for 30 sec. x 1 ☐ each side	hold for 30 sec. x 1 ☐ each side	# lbs _______ # reps _______	# seconds ________

Week 6: Exercise Session #2
Tuesday

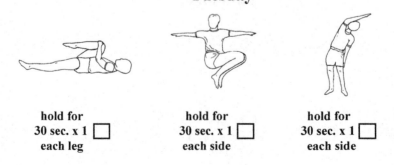

hold for 30 sec. x 1 ☐ each leg	hold for 30 sec. x 1 ☐ each side	hold for 30 sec. x 1 ☐ each side

Week 6: Exercise Session #3
Wednesday

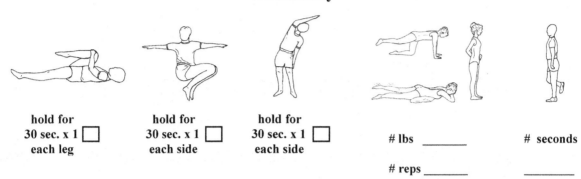

hold for
30 sec. x 1 ☐
each leg

hold for
30 sec. x 1 ☐
each side

hold for
30 sec. x 1 ☐
each side

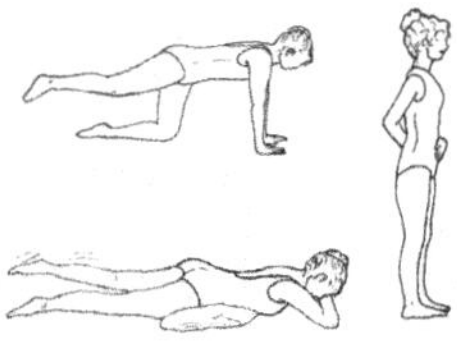

lbs _______

reps _______

seconds

____

Week 6: Exercise Session #4
Thursday

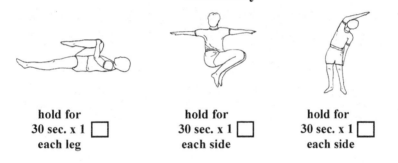

hold for
30 sec. x 1 ☐
each leg

hold for
30 sec. x 1 ☐
each side

hold for
30 sec. x 1 ☐
each side

Week 6: Exercise Session #5
Friday

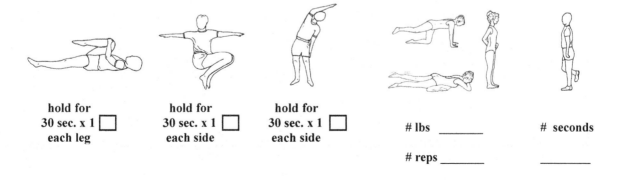

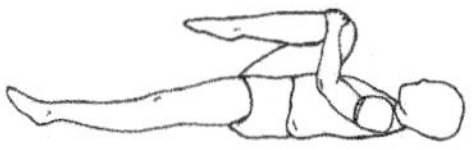

hold for
30 sec. x 1 ☐
each leg

hold for
30 sec. x 1 ☐
each side

hold for
30 sec. x 1 ☐
each side

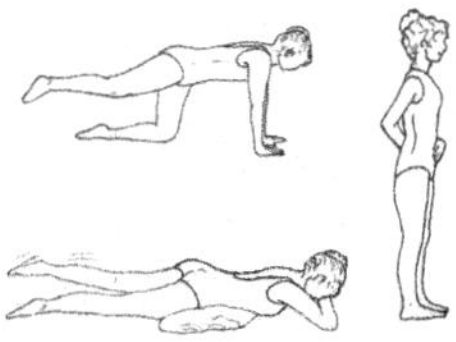

lbs _______

reps _______

seconds

____

Quickstart Guide

- ✓ first, get an okay from your doctor to make sure that the exercises are safe for you to do
- ✓ purchase a pair of adjustable cuff weights if you don't already have them
- ✓ take a look at the six-week plan and pick a day of the week to start
- ✓ on the day you start, it is suggested that you do the exercises in the order pictured, but you don't necessarily *have* to. Use the page numbers provided under each picture to refer to in case you forgot how to do some of the exercises.
- ✓ pick only *one* of the multifidus strengthening exercises that looks comfortable for you to do. Remember to increase the weight when you can do 20 repetitions in good form. Repeat this process to get stronger.
- ✓ use the handy exercise sheets provided to keep track of your workouts
- ✓ try to stick with the routine for at least six weeks for best results

7 Measure Your Progress

Okay. You've learned all about spinal stenosis, started the exercises, and are on the road to recovery. So now what should you expect?

Well, we all know you should expect to get better. But what exactly does *better* mean? As a physical therapist treating patients, it means two distinct things to me:

- your back and legs start to *feel* better

  and

- your back and legs start to *work* better

And so, when a patient returns for a follow-up visit, I will re-assess them, looking for specific changes in their back and leg **pain**, as well as their back and leg **function**.

In this book, I'm going to recommend that readers do the same thing periodically. Why? Simply because people in pain can't always see the progress they're making. For instance, sometimes a person's back and leg pain are exactly the same, but they aren't aware that they can now actually do some motions or tasks that they couldn't do before–a sure sign that things are healing. Or, sometimes a person still has significant back and leg pain, but they're not aware that it's actually occurring less frequently–yet another good indication that positive changes are taking place.

Whatever the case may be, if a person isn't looking at the big picture, and doesn't think they're getting any better, they're likely to get discouraged and stop doing their exercises altogether–even though they really might have been on the right track!

On the other hand though, what if you periodically check your progress and are keenly aware that your back and leg *are* making some changes for the better? What if you can *positively* see objective results? My guess is that you're going to be giving yourself a healthy dose of motivation to keep on truckin' with the exercises.

Having said that, I'm going to show you exactly what to check for from time-to-time so that you can monitor the changes that are taking place. I call them "outcomes" and there are two of them.

Outcome #1:
Look for Changes in Your Pain

First of all, you should look for changes in your pain. I know this may sound silly, but sometimes it's my job to get a person to see that their pain *is* actually improving. You see, a lot of people come to physical therapy thinking they're going to be pain-free right away. Then, when they're not instantly better and still having pain, they often start to worry and become discouraged. Truth is, I have yet to put a patient on an exercise program for spinal stenosis and have them get instantly better. Better yes, but not *instantly* better.

Over the years, I have found that patients usually respond to exercises in a quite predictable pattern. One of three things will almost always occur as patients begin to turn the corner and get better:

- your back and leg pain will be just as intense as always, however now it is occurring much less frequently

or

- your back and leg pain is now *less* intense, even though it is still occurring just as frequently

or

- you start to notice less intense back and leg pain *and* it is now occurring less frequently

The point here is to make sure that you keep a sharp eye out for any of these three changes as you progress with the routines. If *any* of them occur, it will be a sure sign that the exercises are helping. You can then look forward to the pain gradually getting better, usually over the weeks to come.

Outcome #2:
Look for Changes in Back and Leg Function

Looking at how well your back and legs work is very important because many times back function improves *before* the pain does. For example, sometimes a patient will do the exercises for a while, and although their back and leg will still hurt a lot, they are able to do many things that they hadn't been able to in a while–a really good indicator that healing is taking place *and* that the pain should be easing up soon.

While measuring your back and leg function may sound like a pain in the butt, it doesn't have to be. In this book, I'm recommending that readers use a quick and easy assessment tool known as *The Swiss Spinal Stenosis Questionnaire.*

The Swiss Spinal Stenosis Questionnaire has been around for a little while and is very well researched. Studies show that it is a valid test (Stucki 1996, Tomkins 2007), has good test-retest reliability (Stucki 1996, Pratt 2002), and is responsive to clinical changes (Stucki 1996). And best of all, it takes only a couple of minutes to complete. Now that's my kinda test!

So what exactly does taking the Swiss Spinal Stenosis Questionnaire involve? Not much.

- there are two scales on the next two pages
- the first one has seven questions. Answer them by circling the number that best fits your situation. Then, add up the circled numbers and divide by 7 to get your *symptom* score.
- the second scale has five questions. Answer them by circling the number that best fits your situation. Then, add up the circled numbers and divide by 5 to get your *function* score.

The scales that make up the questionnaire are on the pages that follow…

Swiss Spinal Stenosis Questionnaire

Symptom Severity Scale

In the last month, how would you describe ...

The pain you have had on average including pain in your back, buttocks and pain that goes down the legs? (circle a number)

1 None
2 Mild
3 Moderate
4 Severe
5 Very severe

How often have you had back, buttock, or leg pain? (circle a number)

1 Less than once a week
2 At least once a week
3 Everyday, for at least a few minutes
4 Everyday, for most of the day
5 Every minute of the day

The pain in your back or buttocks? (circle a number)

1 None
2 Mild
3 Moderate
4 Severe
5 Very severe

The pain in your legs or feet? (circle a number)

1 None
2 Mild
3 Moderate
4 Severe
5 Very severe

Numbness or tingling in your legs or feet? (circle a number)

1 None
2 Mild
3 Moderate
4 Severe
5 Very severe

Weakness in your legs or feet? (circle a number)

1 None
2 Mild
3 Moderate
4 Severe
5 Very severe

Problems with your balance? (circle a number)

1 No, I've had no problems with balance
3 Yes, sometimes I feel my balance is off, or that I am not sure-footed
5 Yes, often I feel my balance is off, or that I am not sure-footed

Now, add up the circled numbers and divide by 7 to get your score_______

Swiss Spinal Stenosis Questionnaire

Physical Function Scale

In the last month, on a typical day…

How far have you been able to walk? (circle a number)

1 Over 2 miles
2 Over 2 blocks, but less than 2 miles
3 Over 50 feet, but less than 2 blocks
4 Less than 50 feet

Have you taken walks outdoors or in malls for pleasure? (circle a number)

1 Yes, comfortably
2 Yes, but sometimes with pain
3 Yes, but always with pain
4 No

Have you been shopping for groceries or other items? (circle a number)

1 Yes, comfortably
2 Yes, but sometimes with pain
3 Yes, but always with pain
4 No

Have you walked around the different rooms in your house or apartment? (circle a number)

1 Yes, comfortably
2 Yes, but sometimes with pain
3 Yes, but always with pain
4 No

Have you walked from your bedroom to the bathroom? (circle a number)

1 Yes, comfortably
2 Yes, but sometimes with pain
3 Yes, but always with pain
4 No

Now, add up the circled numbers and divide by 5 to get your score_______

*Please note that the Swiss Spinal Stenosis Questionnaire was developed by Dr. Stucki and consists of three scales, two of which are presented here. Also, the original questionnaire does not contain numbers to circle, but they were included here so that the scales could be self-scored.

So how did you do? Keep in mind that with the first set of questions, *the Symptom Severity Scale*, your score will range anywhere from 1 to 5, while the second scale, *the Physical Function Scale*, ranges from 1 to 4. Higher scores mean you're in bad shape, so your goal is to score as *low* as possible.

If you did score high though, don't worry. Just keep taking the questionnaire every few weeks, and as you progress with the exercises, you should see your score go lower and lower as time passes. Remember, sometimes back and leg function gets better *before* the pain does.

Quick Review

- ✓ **being aware of your progress is an important part of treating your spinal stenosis–it motivates you to keep doing the exercises.**
- ✓ **look for the pain to become less *intense*, less *frequent*, or both to let you know that the exercises are helping**
- ✓ **sometimes your back and legs start to work better *before* they start to feel better. Taking *The Swiss Spinal Stenosis Questionnaire* from time-to-time makes you aware of improving pain, as well as back and leg function.**

8 Comprehensive List of Supporting References

Well, we've come a long way since page one. Now that we're coming to the end, I'd like to take a few minutes out to show you all the research that went into this book.

The following is a list of all the randomized controlled trials and scientific studies that have been published in peer-reviewed journals that this book is based on. To make a long story short, there's no nonsense going on here–*every* piece of information you've just read has a good evidence-based reason for being here!

Having said that, I've included this handy reference section so that readers can check out the information for themselves if they wish. Good luck!

Chapter 1

Boden S, et al. Abnormal magnetic-resonance scans of the lumbar spine in asymptomatic subjects. *Journal of Bone and Joint Surgery* 1990;72-A:403-8.

Boos N, et al. The diagnostic accuracy of magnetic resonance imaging, work perception, and psychosocial factors in identifying symptomatic disc herniations. *Spine* 1995;20:2613-2625.

Butler D, et al. Discs degenerate before facets. *Spine* 1990;15:111-113.

Haig A, et al. Electromyographic and magnetic resonance imaging to predict lumbar stenosis, low-back pain, and no back symptoms. *The Journal of Bone and Joint Surgery* 2007;89-A:358-366.

Hitselberger W, et al. Abnormal myelograms in asymptomatic patients. *J Neurosurg* 1968;28:204-6.

Kirkaldy-Willis WH, et al. Pathology and pathogenesis of lumbar spondylosis and stenosis. *Spine* 1978;3:319-328.

Tong H, et al. Magnetic resonance imaging of the lumbar spine in asymptomatic older adults. *Journal of Back and Musculoskeletal Rehabilitation* 2006;19:67-72.

Weishaupt D, et al. MR imaging of the lumbar spine: prevalence of intervertebral disk extrusion and sequestration, nerve root compression, end plate abnormalities, and osteoarthritis of the facet joints in asymptomatic volunteers. *Radiology* 1998;209:661-666.

Yagci I, et al. The utility of lumbar paraspinal mapping in the diagnosis of lumbar spinal stenosis. *Am J Phys Med Rehabil* 2009;88:843-851.

Chapter 2

Amundsen T, et al. Lumbar spinal stenosis: conservative or surgical management? *Spine* 2000;25:1424-36.

Arokoski J, et al. Back and hip extensor muscle function during therapeutic exercises. *Arch Phys Med Rehabil* 1999;80:842-850.

Haig A, et al. Predictors of pain and function in persons with spinal stenosis, low back pain, and no back pain. *Spine* 2006;31:2950-57.

Herno A, et al. Lumbar spinal stenosis; a matched-pair study of operated and non-operated patients. *British Journal of Neurosurgery* 1996;10:461-465.

Johnsson K, et al. The natural course of lumbar spinal stenosis. *Clinical Orthopaedics and Related Research* 1992;279:82-86.

Chapter 3

Berger R, et. al. Effect of various repetitive rates in weight training on improvements in strength and endurance. *J Assoc Phys Mental Rehabil* 1966;20:205-207.

Braith R, et. al. Comparison of 2 vs 3 days/week of variable resistance training during 10- and 18- week programs. *Int J Sports Med* 1989;10:450-454.

Carroll T, et. al. Resistance training frequency: strength and myosin heavy chain responses to two and three bouts per week. *Eur J Appl Physiol* 1998;78:270-275.

DeMichele P, et. al. Isometric torso rotation strength: effect of training frequency on its development. *Arch Phys Med Rehabil* 1997;78:64-69.

Ekstrom R, et al. Surface electromyographic analysis of the low back muscles during rehabilitation exercises. *J Orthop Sports Phys Ther* 2008;38:736-45.

Ekstrom R, et al. Electromyographic analysis of core trunk, hip, and thigh muscles during 9 rehabilitation exercises. *J Orthop Sports Phys Ther* 2007;37:754-62.

Esquivel A, et al. High and low volume resistance training and vascular function. *Int J of Sports Med* 2007;28:217-221.

Hass C, et. al. Single versus multiple sets in long-term recreational weightlifters. *Medicine and Science in Sports and Exercise* 2000;32:235-242.

Hides J, et al. Multifidus muscle recovery is not automatic after resolution of acute, first-episode low back pain. *Spine* 1996;21:2763-69.

Leinonen V, et al. Paraspinal muscle denervation, paradoxically good lumbar endurance, and an abnormal flexion-extension cycle in lumbar spinal stenosis. *Spine* 2003;28:324-331.

O'Shea P. Effects of selected weight training programs on the development of strength and muscle hypertrophy. *Research Quarterly* 1966;37:95-102.

Palmieri G. Weight training and repetition speed. *Journal of Applied Sport Science Research* 1987;1:36-38.

Reid C, et. al. Weight training and strength, cardiorespiratory functioning and body composition of men. *Br J Sports Med* 1987;21:40-44.

Silvester L, et. al. The effect of variable resistance and free-weight training programs on strength and vertical jump. *Natl Strength Cond J* 1982;3:30-33.

Starkey D, et. al. Effect of resistance training volume on strength and muscle thickness. *Medicine and Science in Sports and Exercise* 1996;28:1311-1320.

Stevens V, et al. Electromyographic activity of trunk and hip muscles during stabilization excercises in four-point kneeling in healthy volunteers. *Eur Spine J* 2007;16:711-718.

Stowers T, et. al. The short-term effects of three different strength-power training methods. *Natl Strength Cond J* 1983;5:24-27.

Yagci I, et al. The utility of lumbar paraspinal mapping in the diagnosis of lumbar spinal stenosis. *Am J Phys Med Rehabil* 2009;88:843-851.

Young W, Bilby G. The effect of voluntary effort to influence speed of contraction on strength, muscular power, and hypertrophy development. *J of Strength and Conditioning Research* 1993;7:172-178.

Chapter 4

Bandy W, et. al. The effect of static stretch and dynamic range of motion training on the flexibility of the hamstring muscles. *Journal of Orthopaedic and Sports Physical Therapy* 1998;27:295-300.

Bandy W, et. al. The effect of time and frequency of static stretching on flexibility of the hamstring muscles. *Physical Therapy* 1997;77:1090-1096.

Bandy W, Irion J. The effect of time on static stretch on the flexibility of the hamstring muscles. *Physical Therapy* 1994;74:845-852.

Iversen M, et al. Pilot case control study of postural sway and balance performance in aging adults with degenerative lumbar spinal stenosis. *Journal of Geriatric Physical Therapy* 2009;32:15-21.

McGregor A, et al. Quantitative assessment of the motion of the lumbar spine in the low back population and the effect of different spinal pathologies on this motion. *Eur Spine J* 1997;6:308-315.

Chapter 5

Burton A. Trunk muscle activity induced by three sizes of wobble (balance) boards. *Journal of Orthopaedic and Sports Physical Therapy* 1986;8:27-29.

Leinonen V, et al. Impaired lumbar movement perception in association with postural stability and motor- and somatosensory-evoked potentials in lumbar spinal stenosis. *Spine* 2002;27:975-83.

Chapter 6

Koc Z, et al. Effectiveness of physical therapy and epidural steroid injections in lumbar spinal stenosis. *Spine* 2009;34:985-989.

Chapter 7

Pratt R, et al. The reliability of the Shuttle Walking Test, the Swiss Spinal Stenosis Questionnaire. The Oxford Spinal Stenosis Score, and the Oswestry Disability Index in the assessment of patients with lumbar spinal stenosis. *Spine* 2002;27:84-91.

Stucki G, et al. Measurement properties of a self-administered outcome measure in lumbar spinal stenosis. *Spine* 1996;21:796-803.

Tomkins, C, et al. Construct validity of the physical function scale of the Swiss Spinal Stenosis Questionnaire for the measurement of walking capacity. *Spine* 2007;32:1896-1901.

CPSIA information can be obtained
at www.ICGtesting.com
Printed in the USA
BVOW04s0006220717
489695BV00002B/7/P

9 781457 540189